MEDICINE
through the ages

PETER MANTIN RICHARD PULLEY

610·9

Stanley Thornes (Publishers) Ltd

Originally published in 1988 by Hutchinson Education
Reprinted 1988

Reprinted in 1989 by
Stanley Thornes (Publishers) Ltd
Old Station Drive
Leckhampton
CHELTENHAM GL53 0DN

Reprinted 1990

British Library Cataloguing in Publication Data

Mantin, Peter
   Medicine through the ages.
   1. Medicine—History
   I. Title   II. Pulley, Richard
   610'.9   R131
   ISBN 0 7487 0268 7

Set in Times and Helvetica

Printed and bound in Great Britain at
The Bath Press, Avon

To our pupils past and present

We would like to thank the following for their help with this book:

Typing: J Bishop
Research: J Howard and S Hiscock
Artwork advice: J Greatorex
Photography: G Greatorex

Contents

To the teacher

The book is divided into four sections, which cover the areas included in the GCSE examination.

The first section is a **chronological survey** of medical developments. For each period there is a 'way of life' unit, giving the historical background, followed by a unit on the medical developments in that period.

The second section covers the major **themes** in the history of medicine, making connections through time, as required by the examinations.

The third section looks at **factors of change**, making the shift from asking what happened, to considering why it happened, and covering the main conceptual aspects of the course.

Finally, the **revision section** unites the major ideas that pupils need for the examination, presenting them with exercises which test the range of skills needed for GCSE. Particular emphasis has been laid on **study skills**, asking pupils to refer back to the rest of the book to find and select appropriate evidence to support their answers. You may also want to use parts of this section to check and test **comprehension** of earlier parts of the course.

Every unit poses **questions about the evidence** and narrative in the double-page spread, but also offers more challenging questions about the value and usefulness of the evidence and about the links which may be made with other parts of the book. This makes pupils more aware of the need both to make and explain connections. A **wordbox** in many units helps pupils to understand vocabulary in context.

The whole book is divided into double-page spreads for *easy reference*, so that teachers can relate chronology, themes and factors in the most appropriate way for their own groups and teaching styles. You may want to get the outline chronology clear before you move on to themes and factors, or you may want to break off from the narrative background to slot in appropriate parts of the themes or factors. The structure of the book gives you the **flexibility** you need.

To the student

This book is intended to help you pass your GCSE History examination. You will need to know not only about medicine but also about how we know and write about the past. So you will be asked questions in the book about what you have learned and how you found it out. We use **evidence** to find out about the past, so it is important to understand that it can be used in a variety of ways. This book helps you find out about the history of medicine, by looking at some of the evidence.

History is not only about evidence. It is also about the way in which things **change.** There are many different ways of looking at change – it may be fast, slow, for the better or for the worse. So in the first section of the book we will be looking at **medicine through time**, examining the way of life of different civilizations and seeing how medicine changed over the years. The story will be brought right up to date, looking at some important medical problems affecting us now and perhaps in the future.

The second section looks at **themes**. These are important areas of medicine which can be better understood when seen across different periods. So this will involve examining how different civilizations – such as the Greeks, Romans etc – dealt with the same problem, for example, surgery.

We do not need just to understand how things change. If we are to make sense of the past we need to understand why things change. These things are called **factors**. We will be looking at different factors, such as war, government, religion, and seeing how they affect medicine. Sometimes these factors help the progress of medical knowledge, but on other occasions they hold it back.

The final revision section has been included to help you check your knowledge, and to bring together some of the different ideas you have been studying. You will be given exercises and problems which have been designed to help you answer examination questions. This will involve finding examples from the history of medicine and using them to explain your answers.

Prehistoric medicine

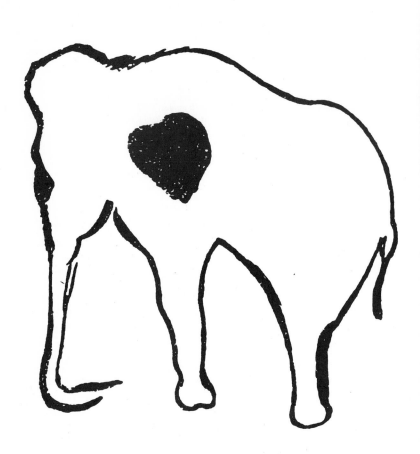

A Cave painting from El Pindal, Spain.

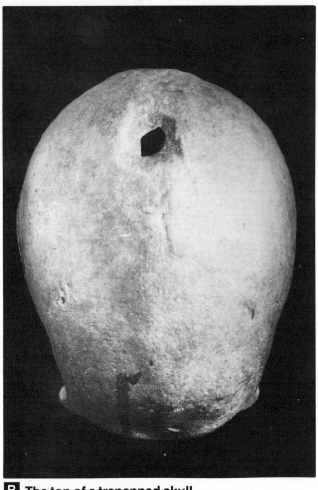

B The top of a trepanned skull.

Prehistory is the time before we have written evidence or proof. It is not easy to find out about medicine in prehistoric times because we don't have much evidence to work with. Archaeologists – people who dig up evidence about the past – have found clues which tell us something about medicine in prehistoric times, but much of the evidence is missing and some of the clues are difficult to make sense of. Look at the following pieces of evidence and see what you can work out about early man's ideas about medicine.

Masks like the ones shown in picture **C** can tell us something about the medical ideas of the people who made them.

D From Dan McKenzie, 'The Infancy of Medicine'.

"

When someone from the Dyak tribe of Borneo is seized with vomiting and sweating, he thinks that an unfriendly ancestral spirit has chased out his soul and has taken its place. So he sends for a wise woman . . . and after she has identified the intruding spirit . . . a doll is moulded from the ashes of the hearth, and . . . the wise woman moves it seven times up and down before the patient. Then the patient spits on the doll, and the disease is transferred to the spirit through the doll.

"

6

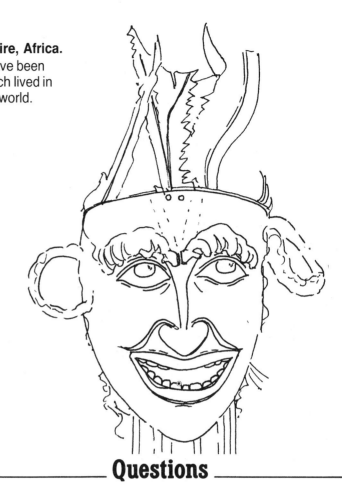

C **Carved and painted wooden masks from Zaire, Africa.**
Similar types of masks have been found amongst tribes which lived in very different parts of the world.

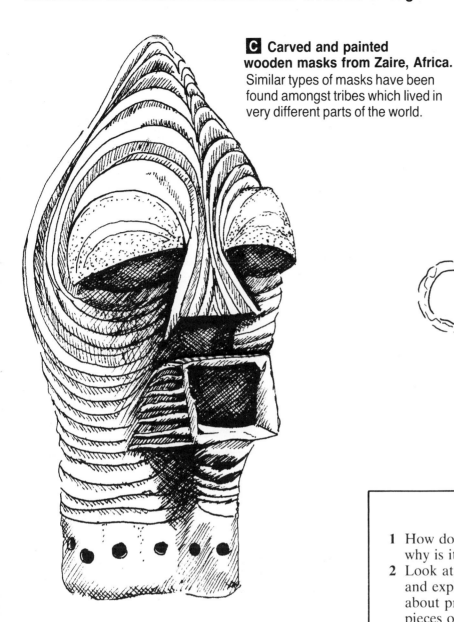

E Jonathan Miller, 'The Body in Question', 1978.
This passage describes the experience of an English scientist who went to live among the Azande tribe of Africa in the 1920s.

"

He was struck by their attitude to physical illness. Whenever members of the tribe felt seriously ill they almost always said it was caused by the bad feelings of friends, relatives or neighbours. No attempt was made to establish the identity of the illness but they consulted a witch doctor to find out who was harming them.

"

Questions

1 How do we know about prehistoric medicine and why is it so hard to find out about it?
2 Look at **A** and **B**. Then copy out these sentences and explain what we might be able to work out about prehistoric medicine from each of these pieces of evidence.
   a The cave painting shows the animal's heart.
   b A lot of skulls have been found with holes drilled in them.
   c In lots of the skulls the bone had grown again after the hole had been drilled.
   d Sharp and pointed antlers of stags were found near many of the skulls.
3 Read documents **D** and **E**. What similarity do you notice in the way these tribes understood:
   a what caused disease, and
   b how disease could be cured?
4 The tribes mentioned in documents **D** and **E** lived far away from each other – in different continents – yet they had very similar ideas about medicine. How do you explain this?

The aborigines

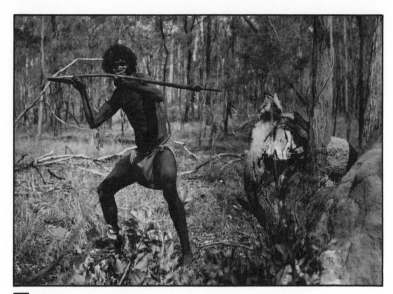

A A modern aborigine using traditional hunting equipment and methods.

The aborigines of Australia are of great interest to historians. Their way of life has changed very little over many centuries. As recently as 100 years ago they used only stone tools, and even today many of their customs and traditions survive. Studying the remaining aborigines may reveal much about other societies that no longer exist.

Geography
Aborigines in the past lived in the desert in hot, hostile, unpleasant conditions. There wasn't much vegetation, and life was a struggle for survival. The aborigines had to live close to nature.

Economy
Photograph **A** gives us clues about the skills the aborigines had, the way they got their food and the kind of life they lived.

Technology
The aborigines had stone tools and weapons. They could build shelters but did not need complicated buildings, as they had to move often, from place to place, in search of food. They used boomerangs, arrows and spears, but lived such a simple life that only simple technology was necessary or possible.

Government
They lived in small groups. The land could not support a large population; there was no main government or leader. Men had most of the power.

Thinking
Aborigines did not read or write and had little technology. They used spirits, gods and mythical stories to explain the world they didn't understand. Spirits created the world, were everywhere and in everything. Their spirit stories were mostly to do with animals – not surprising since they lived so close to nature. Indeed, they saw themselves as members of the animal kingdom. The Kangaroo Man made the gum trees, the Sun Man made the lakes and the Rainbow Serpent made the rivers.

The medicine of the aborigines
Aborigines believed there were good spirits and bad spirits. Most of the time the good spirits looked after the tribe because of the activities (dancing, chanting) of the medicine man. The medicine man got all his power from the spirit world, which he said he alone could fully understand. Through dancing, chanting and picture making he got in touch with the spirits and got their help to heal the sick. The medicine man was as respected as the chief. He was a mixture of priest, doctor and artist.

The medicine man did not really have the same sort of skills as a doctor today, but he was accepted as a healer. If he ever failed it was not the medicine man's fault but the fault of the patient who had upset the spirits or, perhaps, the spirits were too strong to be stopped. All this made good sense to the aborigines, particularly when we remember the way they lived.

These hunters felt at home with nature. They saw themselves as part of a world made up not

Questions

1 Can we study the way of life of people like the aborigines to find out about prehistoric medicine?
2 Look at photograph **A**. Explain how the aborigines got their food and describe the skills they needed to survive in such difficult conditions.
3 The aborigines had no contact with the outside world. Do you think this was:
  a an advantage for aborigine medicine, or
  b a disadvantage for aborigine medicine?
4 **a** What did the aborigines think caused disease?
  b Where do you think the aborigines got this idea about the cause of disease from?
5 How do you think the aborigines' hunting and survival skills helped them with their medicine?

only of plants and animals, but also of spirits, who were just as alive as they were. To the hunter, illness was a natural part of life, from which, through the aid of spirits, people could recover.

Some of the problems that the medicine man had to deal with were simple. These could be treated with things from the world of nature. For example, broken arms were set with mud, burns were treated with sap from trees, stomach pains were dealt with by chewing orchid bulbs, and cuts were covered with animal fat and bound with kangaroo skin.

However, diseases which had no obvious physical cause could not be explained so easily. These diseases were said to be caused by evil spirits and needed special treatment by the medicine man.

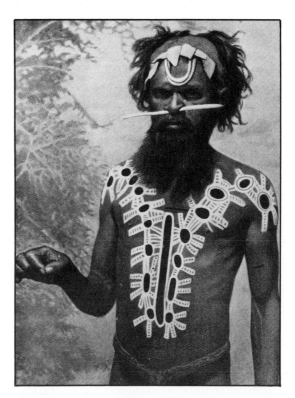

B *(Right)* **Australian aborigine medicine man with healing crystal.**

C *(Below)* **An Australian aborigine medicine man curing his patient.**

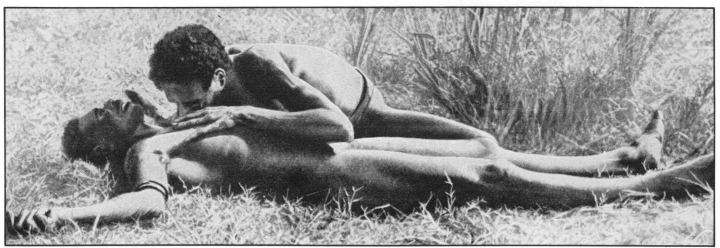

Questions

6 Give examples of medical problems for which the aborigines might go to the medicine man for treatment.

7 The medicine men didn't know about science, but their treatments were often successful. How do you explain this?

8 Why might it make sense to the aborigine to lie down and wait to die if the medicine man refused to treat him?

9 If some of the medicine man's treatments obviously didn't work, why did patients carry on going to him for treatment?

10 Use the information on these two pages to describe what a visit to a medicine man might have been like. Describe what was wrong with you, how the medicine man treated you and why he used those methods.

Ancient Egypt - the way of life

Even though the Egyptian civilization began over 3000 years ago, we can find out a lot about it because the Egyptians left so much evidence behind. Carvings on monuments and paintings found on tomb walls give us valuable clues about the way the Egyptians lived and the things in which they believed.

Geography

Like the aborigines, many Egyptians lived in hot, hostile desert conditions. The big difference was, however, that the Egyptians were able to make use of the River Nile. Many great civilizations grew up near rivers. Map **A** shows the Nile and the huge empire that was conquered as a result of controlling the river.

Economy

The Egyptians got their food in a different way from the aborigines. Picture **B** gives us clues about the skills the Egyptians had and the way in which they organized the work. It was the way in which they made use of the River Nile which allowed the Egyptians to have such a different lifestyle from the aborigines. The economy depended on the way the Egyptians organized the workers, shown in the pictures on this page.

Government

The Egyptians, with their settled way of life, began to build cities, such as Thebes. Many of the temples and houses were built of stone and have survived to this day. With many people to organize and a large empire to control, a powerful government was needed. The pharaoh had absolute control and was worshipped as a god. Picture **D** gives clues about the way this power could be used and helps us understand how the huge empire shown in map **A** had been conquered and its peoples controlled.

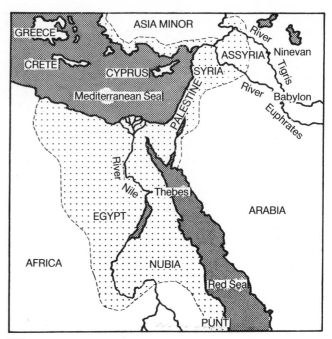

A The Egyptian empire and the River Nile.

B *(Below)* A wall painting from an Egyptian tomb.

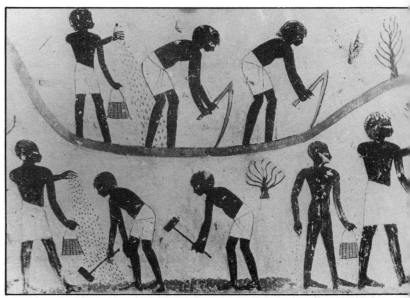

Wordbox

Pharaoh king, ruler
hieroglyphics picture writing

Questions

1 Why do you think the River Nile was so important to the Egyptians?

2 Use picture **B** to explain how the Egyptians got much of their food.

3 Use pictures **B** and **D** to explain how the Egyptian pharaohs used their power. How do you think they kept huge numbers of slave workers under control?

4 List some ways in which religion affected the way of life of the Egyptians.

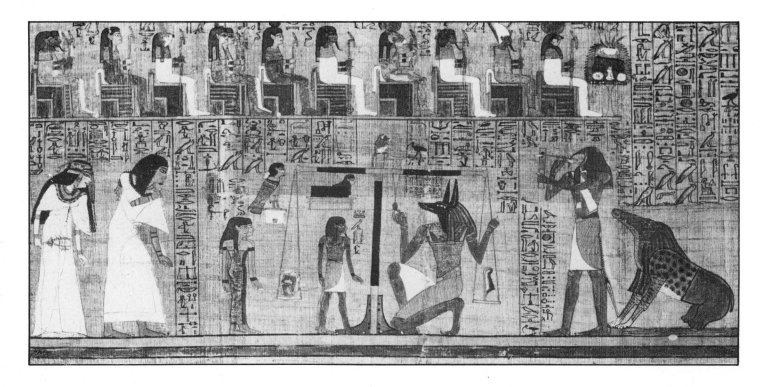

C 'The weighing of the heart and the feather' from 'The Book of the Dead'.

Thinking

The Egyptians had time to learn to read and write. Their beautiful hieroglyphic picture writing can be seen in the picture above. Writing was very important to the Egyptians. They drew picture stories which tell us about their religious ideas. We know that they believed in life after death but can you work out what's happening in picture **C** ? They explained their world in terms of gods and worshipped the sun. Humans were said to have been made at a potter's wheel by the god Khum.

Almost everything in the Egyptians' world had something to do with religion. Huge pyramids were built in which the pharaohs were buried and massive treasures were collected to be buried for use in the next world. Huge statues of the god-like pharaohs were built (see picture **D**).

Generations of men lived and died building these colossal structures.

Technology

The Egyptians learned how to make and use bronze tools; these were an improvement on stone implements. Picture **B** shows vital pieces of farming technology. Look at any of their pictures, paintings and carving and you can get some idea of their skills.

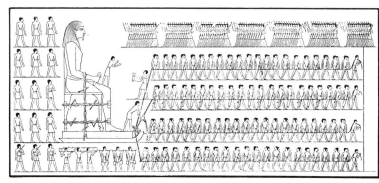

D 'Moving the statue' – a tomb painting.

Questions

5 Give reasons why it is easier to find out about the Egyptians' way of life than that of the aborigines.

6 Compare Egyptian and aborigine technology (see page 8). What differences do you notice?

7 From what you know about the Egyptians' way of life, would you expect their medicine to be similar to or different from that of the aborigines? Give as many reasons as you can for your answer.

Ancient Egypt - medicine

Use the information in this unit to compare Egyptian medicine with Stone Age and aborigine medicine. Look for areas of medicine that have either changed or stayed the same and try to find evidence of scientific or superstitious ideas.

Scientific knowledge existed alongside religious and superstitious ideas in ancient Egypt. Egyptians believed that the war goddess Sekhmet caused and cured epidemics. They believed that a nasty god called Bes might frighten away evil spirits. They worshipped animals and kept lucky scarab beetle charms to scare away evil spirits.

Because the priests spoke to the gods, and because the gods caused disease, it is understandable that the priests should have been involved with medicine. They became healers and physicians and encouraged health and cleanliness. They spread belief in a life after death and encouraged loyalty to and worship of the pharaoh. The body of a pharaoh was mummified in preparation for the next world, but the body organs were cut out and preserved separately.

Jars like those in photograph **B** contained the liver, lungs, stomach and intestines of the person who was going to the next world. Great skill was needed to cut out and preserve the organs of the body. Chemicals like liquid natron, as well as drugs and spices, were needed. The Egyptians got herbs, spices and drugs from all over the middle east and picked up new ideas about medicine from the people with whom they traded.

The embalmers had to be clean and skilful. Some of the Egyptians' drugs, such as opium, castor oil and turpentine are still used today. The Egyptians gave names to the internal organs of the body but because these organs would be needed in the next world, they were not to be cut up.

C Description of the Egyptian 'Code of Hygiene' by Herodotus, a Greek traveller visiting Egypt in the 5th century BC.

"

They are especially religious – more than any other nation; and these are some of their customs. They drink from cups of bronze which they clean daily and this is done not just by some people but by everyone. They are especially careful always to wear newly washed linen clothing. Their priests shave the whole body every third day so that no lice . . . may infest them while they are in the service of the gods . . . Twice a day and every night they wash in cold water.

"

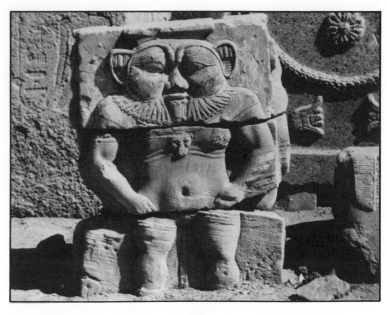

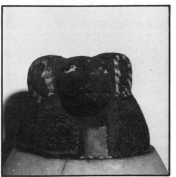

A *(Above)* **The ancient Egyptian god Bes, from the temple of Dendera, Egypt.**

B *(Left)* **The lid of an Egyptian canopic jar used for storing items for the 'after life'.**

Ideas about the cause of disease

Egyptians thought the body was a bit like the River Nile. They used the River Nile for watering their crops. Irrigation channels carried this water and sometimes they got blocked. Egyptians believed the body could also get 'blocked'. To make you better, you had to get 'unblocked' by taking laxatives, vomiting or having bad blood sucked out of you by little black leeches. By looking carefully at the way nature worked Egyptians tried to improve the way in which they looked after their bodies.

We know from well mended fractures found on the limbs of Egyptian mummies that priest physicians looked after their patients well. They could carry out simple, external surgical operations, like cutting out tumours and boils. But they couldn't do more complicated internal operations. They didn't have anaesthetics and they didn't know that the blood circulated around the body. Documents **D**, **E** and **F** tell us more about the Egyptians.

D Recipe from Ebers Papyrus.

" . . . for driving away all kinds of spells. Get a large beetle. Cut its head and wings off, heat its head and wings, lay it in snake's fat, heat it and drink it. "

E Found on a papyrus scroll.

" Remedy for blindness – 'Take a pig's eye, red ochre and a little honey. Mix them and pour into the ear. Then chant a spell . . .' "

F From a report on excavations at Akhetaton in Egypt, carried out by the archaeologist Professor T E Peet.

" The town of Akhetaton was built by the pharaoh Akhnaton about 1370 BC. In the house of the nobleman Nakht was found a bathroom with a drain. There was also a stand for water jars for drinking and washing. Each house in the workmen's village contained four rooms, but there was no evidence of hygienic convenience. Cleanliness was, it seemed, only for the noble, the priest and the official. The workmen's houses were crowded into a small space. "

Wordbox

embalmers people who preserve bodies
irrigation supplying the land with water

anaesthetics something that removes feeling in order to prevent pain
papyrus paper made from reeds

Questions

1 Copy and complete the chart shown. Work out the answers from the information on aborigine and Egyptian medicine. Give examples to back up your answers. Leave enough space to explain each answer in detail.

2 From the chart on this page choose one area of medicine in which great changes took place. Give reasons for these changes.

3 List the ways in which Egyptian medicine could be described as
   a religious, and
   b scientific.

Comparing aborigine and Egyptian medicine

Aborigines/Stone Age	Questions	Egyptians
	a How much did they know about anatomy (the parts of the body)?	
	b How much did they know about physiology (how the body works)?	
	c What did they think caused illness?	
	d What did they know about pharmacology (herbs and drugs)?	
	e Did they know about the need for doctors and nurses?	
	f Did they have surgeons and surgical knowledge?	
	g Did they have a public health system (a way of spreading hygiene to all)?	

Ancient Greece - the way of life

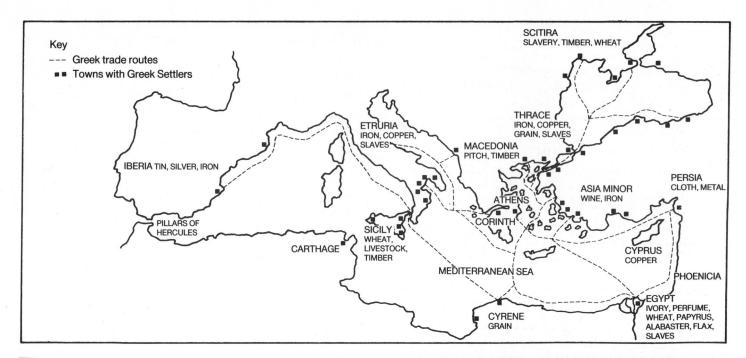

A Ancient Greek settlements and trade routes.

B *(Right)* Greek pottery about 520 BC.

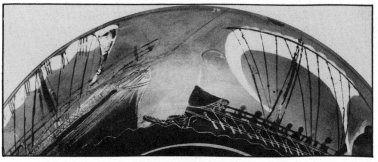

Geography

Map **A** shows the area where the Greeks lived. The climate was warm. Many of the inland areas were hilly, so most of the farming was done on the lowland areas near the coast. Settlements were built along these coastal areas.

Government

Greece wasn't one big country – it was lots of small states. These were called city states. They organized themselves in different ways. Some, called **monarchies**, were ruled by kings. Others, called **democracies**, decided who controlled the city by elections. Others, called **aristocracies**, were ruled by small groups of the richest men. Many of these ways of running a country were copied by other nations later in history.

Economy

The Greeks were able to grow enough food for their needs, and therefore had time left to learn new skills. Pottery, like that shown in picture **B**, has been dug up by archaeologists. It gives us important clues about the Greeks' way of life. The Greeks traded far and wide throughout the Mediterranean and set thousands of slaves to work in the fields, in the home and on building projects like that seen in picture **C**.

Questions

1 Look at Map **A**. Corinth and Athens were two of the most important Greek city states. Name four groups of people they traded with and what items they traded.
2 Give two reasons why you think trade was so important to Greek medicine.
3 Picture **B** shows Greek ships.
   a What differences do you notice between the ships?
   b Why do you think the Greeks needed different types of ships? (Map **A** may help you answer this question.)
4 a The Greeks were ruled in different ways. Name three of them.
   b Which of these three ways of ruling was most like the way in which ancient Egypt was run? Explain your answer.

Thinking

The Greeks believed in a world of many gods. These gods had power to do good and to do harm. Everything seemed to be influenced by the gods – and anyone who angered the gods risked punishment by them. Many Greeks explained things like thunder, lightning, earthquakes, the seasons, war and disease in terms of gods. So in this way they were like the Egyptians. Indeed they also built magnificent temples to their gods – like the one seen in picture **C**.

However, what made the Greeks special and so important was that alongside their belief in gods there grew up, in Greece, a new way of looking at the world. This was called philosophy. This word means 'love of wisdom' and the Greek thinkers who found out many wise and important things were known as the philosophers.

When we looked at the Greek economy we saw that controlling thousands of slaves allowed the Greeks the time to educate themselves. They did this so well that they were able to work out a way of understanding things that we might call a scientific way. This involved thinking of an idea and testing out whether the idea worked in an experiment.

This scientific way of working allowed the Greeks to make new discoveries about the way they worked. They made maps of the known world, learned about maths and physics, and some historians have even said that the ideas on which computers are based come from the Greeks. Sometimes they got it wrong – for example, they believed that the planets were connected to the earth by invisible chains. However, the point was that their method – their scientific way of working – was always likely to help them carry on learning new things.

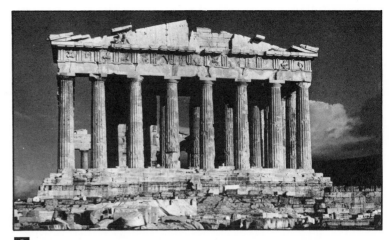

C The ruins of the Parthenon, in Athens, a temple dedicated to the goddess Athena.

Wordbox

monarchy   country or state ruled by a king or queen
democracy   country or state ruled by the group which gets most votes in an election
aristocracy   country or state ruled by a small number of rich people
archaeologists   people who dig up evidence from the past
philosophers   thinkers

Questions

5 From what you know about the Greek way of life would you expect Greek medicine to be more like that of the aborigines or the Egyptians? Explain your answer.

D Summary diagram of the Greek way of life.

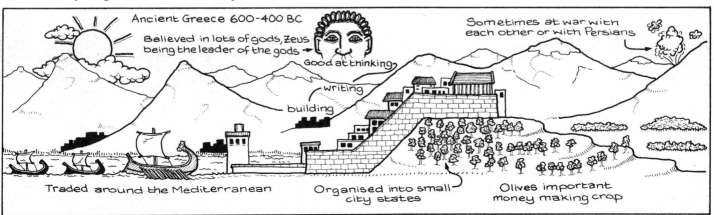

Ancient Greece 600-400 BC

Believed in lots of gods, Zeus being the leader of the gods →

Good at thinking,
writing
building

Sometimes at war with each other or with Persians

Traded around the Mediterranean

Organised into small city states

Olives important money making crop

Ancient Greece - medicine

Like the Egyptians, the Greeks also had a god of healing. He was called Asklepios. Like Imhotep (page 42), Asklepios was probably a physician who lived around 1200 BC. He may have been so successful that his people worshipped him as a god.

Greek legends say that Asklepios healed so many people that the gods became jealous and killed him. Asklepios was said to have had two sons and six daughters, who were all good at healing. One of his daughters, Hygeia, gave her name to the word 'hygienic' – which means 'clean'.

There were temples built in honour of Asklepios in several parts of Greece. People went to these temples to pray to Asklepios in the hope of being cured. The patients told the priest physicians what was wrong with them, and were often cured overnight by his holy snake. Even today the snake is seen on doctors' badges.

C 'Cures by Asklepios', carved on the pillars of the healing temple, or Asklepios, at Epidaurus in Greece.

"

Aristagora had a worm in her belly so she went to the temple. Asklepios was away at the time but his assistant had seen him work, and cut off Aristagora's head. He was unable to put it on again and in the morning saw the head separated from the body. A messenger was sent to the god. Asklepios arrived, put her head back on, opened up her belly, took out the worm, sewed her up again and then she was healed.

A man from Torone drank a mixture of wine and honey into which his evil stepmother had put some leeches; his pain was so great that he had to visit the god Asklepios, who opened his chest with a knife, took out the leeches and sewed up his chest. The man was cured.

"

Questions

1 a What is the god Asklepios doing in the carving? (Picture **A**)
  b How might archaeologists know how to reconstruct Hippocrates' temple? (Picture **B**)
2 From the information on these pages make lists of:
  a Greek scientific ideas, and
  b Greek religious ideas.

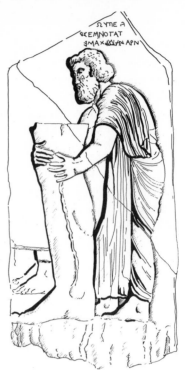

A Stone carving found at the temple of Asklepios.

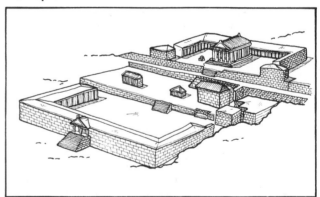

B Reconstruction picture of Hippocrates' temple on Cos.

Greek medicine was made up of lots of ideas, some of which we might call religious and others which could be called scientific. When we looked at the story of Asklepios we saw that the Greeks had a healing god and worshipped him at a temple, which was also a sort of hospital and health resort.

However, scientific Greek doctors put forward the idea that there were natural causes and cures for diseases. The most famous of these doctors was called Hippocrates. He was born on a small Greek island called Cos, in about 460 BC. He was a doctor whose work is known about through a number of medical books that were written about that time. Although these books have been called the Hippocratic Collection, we can't prove that he wrote them. Indeed, some of them were written about 150 years after his death. He is mentioned by two Greek writers, Plato and Aristotle, who lived around the same time. There are lots of statues which are supposed to show what he looked like, but most of them were made after he died.

A large temple of healing, the 'temple of Hippocrates' still stands on Cos, even though part of it is ruined. He was famous enough for people to call him 'The Father of Medicine'. So instead of blaming the gods for illness, the books of doctors like Hippocrates showed how important exercise, diet and fitness were in making the patient feel better. We can see this in the 'Programme for Health'.

D Sections from the 'Programme for Health'.

"

Health begins with the moment a man wakes up. A young or middle-aged man should take a walk of about 10 stadia just before sunrise. (After awakening he should not arise at once but should wait until the heaviness of sleep has gone.) After getting up he should rub the whole body with some oil. Afterwards he should, every day, wash face and eyes with the hands using pure water. He should rub his teeth inside and out with the fingers using some fine peppermint powder and cleaning the teeth of food. He should clean nose and ears inside, preferably with well-perfumed oil. He should rub and clean his head every day but wash it and comb it only at intervals.

After doing these things, people who have to work or choose to work will do so, but rich people will first take a walk. Long walks before meals clear out the body, prepare it for receiving food and give it more power for digesting.

A wise man should remember that health is the greatest of human blessings. In winter, people should eat as much as possible and drink as little as possible – unwatered wine, bread, roast meat and few vegetables. This will keep the body hot and dry. In summer they should drink more and eat less – watered wine, barley cakes and boiled meat so that the body will stay cold and moist. Walking should be fast in winter and slow in summer.

"

The Greeks tried to live as healthily as possible. This is suggested by the fact that they held lots of sports meetings, the most famous of which was the Olympic Games, held every four years at Olympia.

After the collapse of the Greek way of life, the Games seem to have died out. They were brought back only in 1896. It's only in the last century that national sports leagues, international sports fixtures, PE in schools etc. have really grown. Yet thousands of years ago, in ancient Greece, we find detailed reports about PE lessons for pupils, and descriptions of baths, showers and massages for rich people.

Wordbox

stadia measurements of about 200 metres
Olympia a city state in Greece
city state a city which governs itself

Questions

3 Compare Greek medicine with Egyptian medicine. What changes had taken place? Explain your answer.

4 We know the Greeks (or the rich ones) were often fit, strong and healthy. So *why* was Supergreek so big and strong? (Supergreek is in picture **E**.)
Read document **D** again. Next to each box in picture **E** copy a line from document **D** that gives an example of their treatments; e.g. FOOD IN WINTER: 'In winter, people should eat as much as possible and drink as little as possible – unwatered wine, bread, roast meat and few vegetables.'

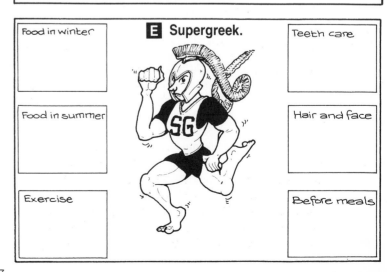

Food in winter — Teeth care — Food in summer — Hair and face — Exercise — Before meals

E Supergreek.

Ancient Rome - the way of life

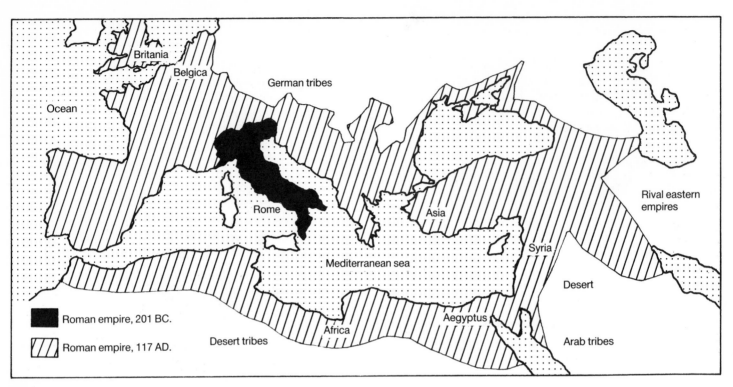

A The Roman empire, from 201 BC to 117 AD. The place names are of Roman provinces.

Geography

The Roman empire lasted for almost 500 years. It included millions of people, from a wide range of different tribes and races, who usually co-operated with the Romans. At the heart of the empire lay Rome, which was the largest city of its time. It was said that all roads led to Rome. The empire can be seen on map **A**.

Government

By 31 BC Rome was ruled by an emperor who took all the decisions without having to ask for anyone's agreement. The army was very important to the Romans, but it was very expensive and so taxes had to be collected from all the people who worked in the empire. Usually the poorer people had to pay the most tax, and it was spent not only on the army but on some of the large public building works like those seen in picture **B**.

To make everything work properly there were lots of government officials who made sure that taxes were duly collected and that towns and cities worked well. Some were involved in the law, and it was said that if you were a free person you could expect the fairest of treatment under it. Historians tell us how the Romans treated conquered peoples.

Livy, a Roman historian, wrote: 'Of the 10,000 free men captured, the Roman commander Scipio released those who were citizens of New Carthage but decided that 2000 craftsmen . . . were to become slaves to the Roman people.'

Josephus, a Jewish historian, wrote about the Roman victory over the Jews: 'Of the Jewish captives, those over seventeen years of age were either chained or sent to labour in the mines of Egypt or were assigned to Asia Minor to die in the amphitheatres, slaughtered by the sword or torn to pieces by wild beasts.'

Economy

The Romans got rich through farming. The mild climate and well organized farms meant that there were lots of crops or livestock to trade around the Mediterranean. By 44 BC Rome was in control of most of the trade in all sorts of goods all over Europe. Trade was not only in farm products but in pottery, glass and metal work.

Technology

We can learn more about Roman skills and technology by looking at evidence they left behind, like that seen in picture **B**.

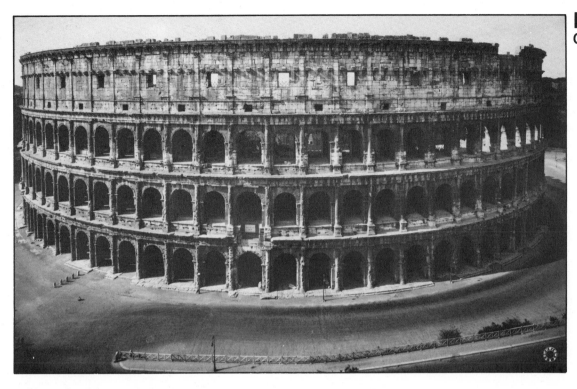

B Remains of the Colosseum, Rome.

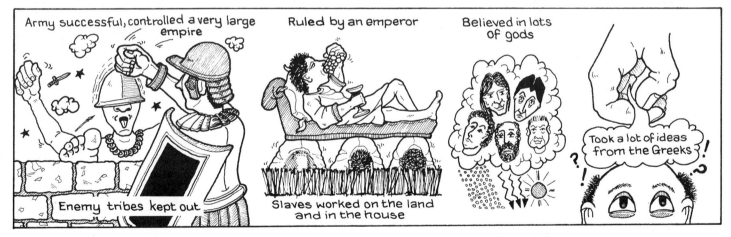

Army successful, controlled a very large empire

Enemy tribes kept out

Ruled by an emperor

Slaves worked on the land and in the house

Believed in lots of gods

Took a lot of ideas from the Greeks

C Summary diagram of the Roman way of life.

Questions

1 Look at map **A**. Use an atlas to list the modern names of countries which were in the Roman empire.
2 The Romans conquered a large empire. Explain how each of the following things helped them: roads, good leaders, the army, taxes, building skills, slaves, farming, trade.
3 The Romans conquered the Greeks. How might this have affected Roman medicine?
4 How could we check to see if Livy or Josephus (the quotations from documents on page 18) is the more reliable historian?

Wordbox

assigned sent
livestock animals
amphitheatre arena or stadium

Ancient Rome - medicine

The Romans did not have many new ideas about the causes or cures of illness. Any ideas they had were mainly taken from the Greeks. They tried to avoid getting ill because they knew that there were few cures. They often turned to gods to heal them. They would go to the temple of Asklepios and make sacrifices to the healing god. He was, as you might remember, well known in ancient Greece and the Romans began to worship him after a bad plague in Rome in 295 BC.

People hoped to see the god in a dream and would talk to the god about their illness. Asklepios might suggest things that would cure them such as bathing, taking herbal remedies, exercise, diet or even writing poetry.

Archaeologists have discovered that people were coming to the temple in Dijon long before Roman times. When the Romans conquered the area it was so popular that they built two temples and a bathing pool. Some of the ways of being cured that they tried might actually have worked, but if they did it would not have been because of any scientific breakthrough but as a result either of people getting over the illness naturally or not being all that ill in the first place. For those with serious complaints there was still no cure.

Even though there were no reliable remedies for illness, some doctors became quite famous in Roman times. One of these was Claudius Galen.

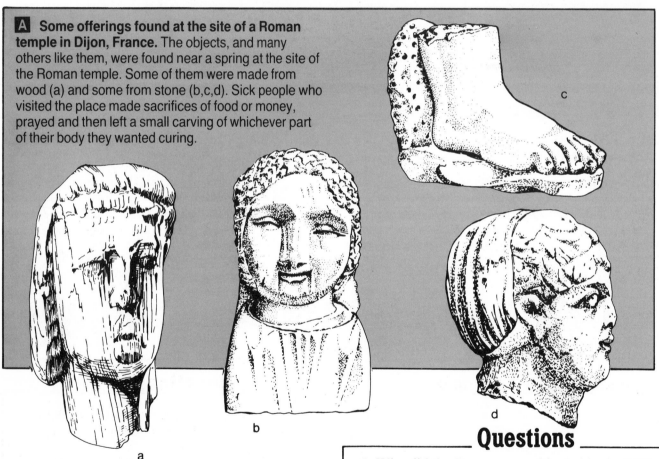

A **Some offerings found at the site of a Roman temple in Dijon, France.** The objects, and many others like them, were found near a spring at the site of the Roman temple. Some of them were made from wood (a) and some from stone (b,c,d). Sick people who visited the place made sacrifices of food or money, prayed and then left a small carving of whichever part of their body they wanted curing.

Wordbox

expanding getting bigger
effectively successfully
phlegm mucus coughed up (it was one of the four humours)
remedies things to make you better

Questions

1 Why did the Romans worship Asklepios? Who else worshipped him?
2 Name two cures Asklepios suggested. Say if you think they would work or not and why they might have been suggested.
3 Look at picture **A**. What might have been wrong with the people who left objects b, c and d?
4 Why do you think the Romans built a temple at Dijon?

Claudius Galen
He was perhaps the most famous doctor of his time and made many important advances in the story of medicine. Galen knew the work of Hippocrates (see page 16) very well and accepted his ideas about the human body being made up of four humours that needed to be kept in balance if people were to stay healthy. He developed this idea by saying that any imbalance in the body caused by a humour expanding and causing illness could be treated effectively by a method called the 'use of opposites'.

This meant that if, for example, someone had a cold caused by too much phlegm they would be encouraged by Galen to eat dry bread or roast meat and if they were to drink anything it must be hot. In other words they would be given the opposite to what seemed to be making them unwell.

Another example might be a fever in summer time when clearly the sufferer would seem to be very hot. Galen would treat this person by suggesting that they eat cool or cold things and that drinking liquids would help them.

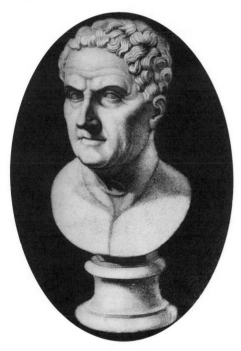

B Claudius Galen from a bust made in Roman times.

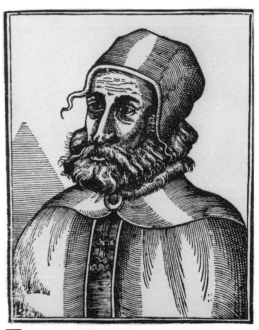

C Cladius Galen, an engraving included in 'Surgery' by Ambroise Paré, 1575.

Questions

5 How reliable do you think picture **C** is as a source of evidence about Galen? Explain your answer.

6 If the bust shown in picture **B** was made before the engraving shown in picture **C**, does this mean that picture **B** is a more reliable source of evidence about Galen's appearance? Explain your answer.

7 Using Galen's idea about the use of opposites, copy the following chart into your books and complete it for all of the seasons. The idea is that you must suggest and draw food that is opposite to the things in the left-hand box. Use the humours diagram to help you (page 44). You should write and draw food you would suggest to a patient ill during this season. It should be opposite to the season. Try to think of Roman type food if you can!

Season	Element	Humour				
WINTER	WATER	PHLEGM	Roast beef	Hot cakes	Hot thick vegetable stew	Onions
			NOW DO THE OTHER THREE SEASONS			

The Middle Ages - the way of life

When we talk about the period of Western history called the Middle Ages, we mean the time from about 500 AD (after the collapse of the Roman Empire) until about 1500 AD. Sometimes historical periods don't have exact beginnings or endings.

Government

During the Middle Ages many of the countries of Europe were organized in what we call today the feudal system. This meant that the people of each country were divided up into different ranks or classes. At the top was the king who gave out land and jobs to the great landowners who in turn gave out land and jobs to others until, at the bottom, there were the peasants. The peasants owned only a very small amount of land.

The great landlords did not always trust or support the king, so kings were not always as powerful as they wanted to be. However, the landlords and the king needed to co-operate to make laws and raise taxes.

Economy

As we see in picture **B**, farming was still an important way to make money; in fact it was the main way. The feudal system did not encourage new ideas to be tried out on the land, and many peasants found it hard to survive the winter and pay their taxes. Unlike Roman times, there was no longer an organized system of slavery. However, we can get an idea of what life was like for peasants when we read the description (document **C**) of conditions in England in the 14th century.

A Extract from 'Piers Ploughman' by William Langland (c 1360).

> The peasants live on milk and oatmeal to make gruel and fill the bellies of their children who cry for food. And they themselves are often starving with hunger. . . Comfort these peasants along with the blind and lame.

Despite the bad roads, trading took place between countries – in woollen cloth, iron, grain, fish and other goods. However, it sometimes took years to make overland journeys to Asia, and ships' captains were not keen to sail far from the sight of land.

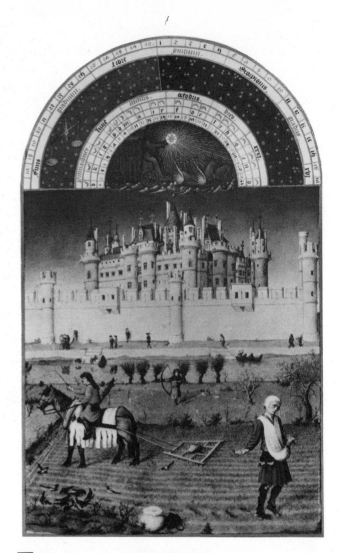

B French painting from the 'Book of Hours', 1413. The painting shows a woman sowing and a man tilling the ground outside a large fortified city. The calendar indicates it is autumn.

Thinking

Christianity had a very big influence on the way in which people understood their world. It did not always encourage new ideas or ways of thinking, but was very important in helping learning. Churches and monasteries collected, copied and wrote books not only about religious things, but also about herbs and medicine, both Greek and Roman.

Wordbox

peasants	poor farmers
dominates	controls by force
slavery	forced working with no pay or freedom

Technology

There were many changes to do with warfare. Both castles and the armour of fighting men became more expensive and complicated. On the land, better quality ploughs were invented (see picture **C**). Windmills and watermills provided power to grind better quality flour. Perhaps the greatest result of the technological advances were the huge cathedrals built all over Europe. The skills needed to design and build them must have been great. However, because books were still written by hand rather than printed, it was not easy to spread knowledge quickly.

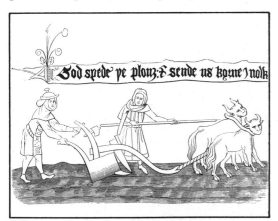

C Ploughing in the Middle Ages.

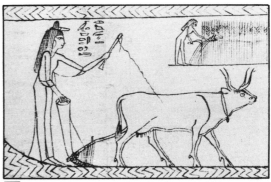

D Egyptian ploughing from the funeral papyrus of Princess Nesitanebtashru, about 970 BC.

Questions

1 Look at pages 22 and 23. Copy the statements below and say whether each is true or false. Give more than one reason for your answer:
   a people knew about science and technology in the Middle Ages,
   b women always worked in the home in the Middle Ages, and
   c under the feudal system, everyone was equal.
2 Look at pictures **C** and **D**. What similarities and differences do you notice between Egyptian and medieval ploughing? Had there been a big change or not? Explain your answer.

3 During the Middle Ages some things changed a lot, other things stayed the same.
   a List the things that changed.
   b List the things that didn't change much.
   c Why might some things change and others stay the same?
4 In this chapter we have looked at paintings, drawings and books from the Middle Ages. What other things might tell us about life in those days? Make a list.
5 Is it easier to find out about medieval kings or medieval peasants? Explain your answer.

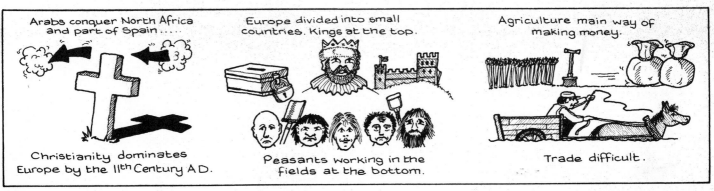

Arabs conquer North Africa and part of Spain.....

Christianity dominates Europe by the 11th Century A.D.

Europe divided into small countries. Kings at the top.

Peasants working in the fields at the bottom.

Agriculture main way of making money.

Trade difficult.

E Summary diagram of the medieval way of life.

The Middle Ages - medicine

A Patricia Morison gives us a modern historian's view of medicine in the Middle Ages. (BBC TV programme 'Timewatch', 1986.)

> Herbs were the foundation of medieval medicine. They were given to rich and poor alike, though how well they worked didn't depend on the size of your purse. You could spend a king's ransom on some fancy eastern recipe and not do any better than with herbs from the local hedgerow. Peasants would have consulted the local wise women who might have been skilled herbalists. However, because they couldn't write we don't know what they prescribed. Doctors, on the other hand-used 'herbals' – books full of hundreds of recipes.
>
> Historians used to dismiss these herbals as nonsense, but latest research on the 'Leech Book' of Bald, an Anglo-Saxon physician, shows that not only was he highly experienced in practical medicine, but that many of his prescriptions were simple, sensible and actually worked. Some, for burns, recommend using butter and eggs, which would have had a soothing effect.

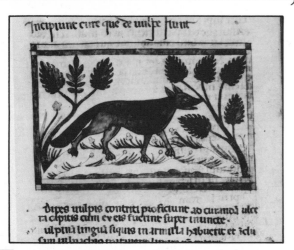

B Pages from a 'herbal' written in the 11th century in Canterbury. The book describes drugs which can be made from animals. The liver and lungs of a fox, finely chopped and taken in wine, were said to be good for asthma.

C From the writing of Cassiodorus, a friend of the monk St Benedict, in the 6th century AD.

> Learn about herbs, and seek to know how to combine the various kinds for human health; do not, however, entirely place your hope on herbs. Since medicine has been created by God, and since it is He who restores health, turn to Him. Do all that you do in word or deed in the name of the Lord Jesus . . . If you cannot read Greek, then read the translations of Hippocrates, Galen and other medical works which, by God's help, I have provided for you in my library.

D A medieval remedy for dysentery, quoted in 'Anglo Saxon Magic' by G. Storms.

> This letter brought by an angel to Rome, when they were sorely afflicted with dysentery. Write this on paper so long that it can go round the head, and hang it on the neck of the man who is in need of it. He will soon be better.

Questions

1 Read document **A**. Did rich and poor get the same medical treatment in the Middle Ages? Explain your answer.
2 Give some reasons why 'wise women' (evidence **A**) did not write books about herbal remedies.
3 Read document **C**. It names *three* things that someone interested in medicine must know about or believe. Say what these three things are and write out the bits of the evidence that gave you the answers.

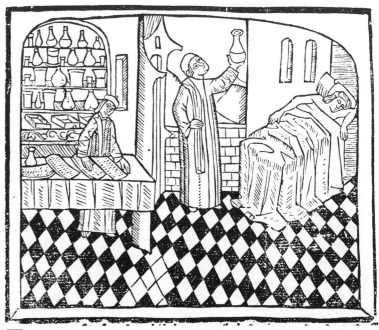

E A doctor treating his patient, 1495.

Before a remedy could be suggested, the doctor had to work out what was wrong. The doctor would look at the patient for signs of sweating, changing skin colour or a change in the pulse. Looking at the colour of urine was often used. Colour charts enabled doctors to work out what was wrong with a patient.

For example, one manuscript from 1506 tells us that: 'Urine red like blood is a sign of fever caused by too much blood . . . Heat is the cause of a red colour, cold of white, dryness is the reason for a thin texture . . .'

The idea that urine could be used to work out an illness comes from the Roman doctor Galen who said: 'the liver generates humours . . . The urine, then, indicates the state of the liver.'

Working out medical problems from urine might present some interesting problems for doctors. For example, Notker was a monk who lived in the 9th century AD. He was said to have performed wonders of healing. There is a story that one of his rich patients, the Duke of Bavaria, wanted to test Notker's skill. Instead of giving him a sample of his own urine the Duke gave Notker urine from a pregnant woman. Notker looked at it and is supposed to have said: 'God is about to perform a miracle. Within 30 days, the Duke will give birth to a child.'

Blood letting

One popular way of treating the sick was a method known as flebotomy. Flebotomy means bleeding. It was done by cutting into veins with knives, by heating small metal cups on the skin and letting them cool.

The people of the Middle Ages were also instructed by doctors to look after their health. Here is some advice from a poem written around the 12th century AD:

'Rise early in the morne, and straight remember,
With water cold to wash your hands and eyes,
Both comb your head, and rub your teeth likewise:
If bled you should keep coole, if bath'd keep warme.'

Wordbox

medieval   of the Middle Ages
foundation   what something is based on
herbalist   someone who knows about herbs
sorely afflicted   had very nasty problems with dysentery
flebotomy   bleeding, or blood letting

F A diagram from a book written in the Middle Ages showing where to bleed people for different illnesses.

Questions

4 What does picture **E** show? Why do you think the doctor is inspecting the bottle?

5 a The black marks on picture **F** are spots of blood. What does this tell you?

   b Look at picture **F**. Blood letting was very dangerous, so why do you think so many people did it?

6 a What similarities and differences do you notice between the way modern doctors work and the way medieval doctors worked?

   b What things did medieval doctors think caused disease?

7 What evidence can you find on these pages to suggest that medieval medicine was based on Greek and Roman ideas?

The Renaissance - the way of life

Historical periods don't always start or finish at convenient dates. The word 'Renaissance' describes a period in European history, but historians cannot agree about when it started or finished. In this book the period we call the Renaissance covers the years 1500-1700.

Renaissance means rebirth. People living during the Renaissance felt that they could recreate and even improve the work of the ancient Greeks and Romans. People also began to challenge some of the ideas of the Middle Ages.

Government

The power of kings and queens began to be challenged by different groups of people, in particular those who had grown rich through trade and business. They wanted more say in matters that affected them. This sometimes led to wars such as the English Civil War (1642–1649).

However, some of the royal families of Europe managed to stay in control of their countries by allowing just a small amount of power to be given to others. These people were wealthy landowners and merchants who could be trusted not to try to take too much control. These newly important people tried to make their countries richer and stronger.

Economy

Many governments during the Renaissance helped businessmen and traders by passing laws to protect and encourage them. So it is not surprising that international trade increased. Merchants began to raise money to help sea captains sail to other countries and trade. Sometimes European countries simply took what they wanted, especially if the people they came into contact with seemed less advanced than Europeans. Examples of this might be the Aztecs of Mexico and the Incas of Peru who were both conquered by the Spanish between 1519 and 1533. Gold, silver and almost everything of value was taken from them.

European merchants with overseas contacts quickly began to grow rich. However, for most of the slowly increasing population of Europe, farming was still the main way of earning a living. For farmers and farm workers this period saw a gradual improvement in their standard of living, which meant that some could afford the goods that resulted from expanding trade.

Technology

This was an age when new inventions were being tried and tested. They would be successful though only if they were quite easy to make, and if they would make some money. Leonardo da Vinci (1452–1519) was one of a number of talented artists working at this time (see picture **B**). As well as painting he invented all kinds of things, including making sketches for tanks and helicopters; but these ideas were too complicated to be made successfully and didn't seem very useful at the time.

One of the most important inventions of this period was the printing press. It was developed in various parts of Europe at about the same time.

Important developments in sailing ships, resulting from a combination of European and Arab technology, made them capable of sailing the world's oceans. Such ships helped Spain and Portugal to build up large overseas empires.

Smaller machines were invented using the skills of watchmakers and clocksmiths. These included the microscope and the telescope. Such instruments were used by people to look in greater detail at the world around them.

A A 16th-century painting called 'The Ambassadors', by Holbein.

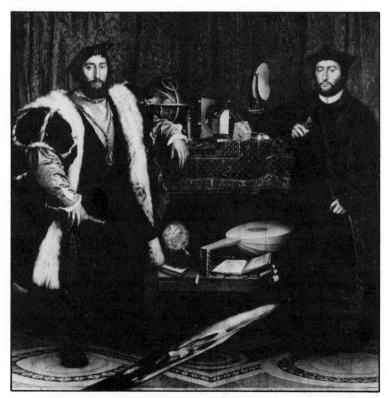

Thinking

Although Christianity still dominated the way that people in Europe thought and acted the Catholic church began to split into different parts or denominations. This change came about because of arguments over how much power the Catholic church should have, and how the Bible should be understood. The rediscovery of the books of Greek and Roman writers and thinkers also encouraged different methods of learning. This resulted in new ideas about art, science, writing and medicine.

Wordbox

recreate   bring to life again or bring back
expanding increasing
dominated controlled

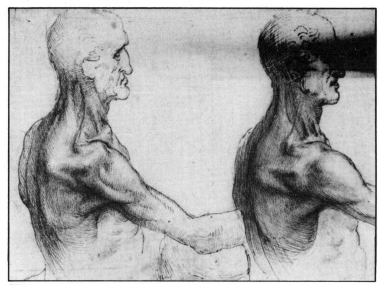
B Drawings by Leonardo da Vinci.

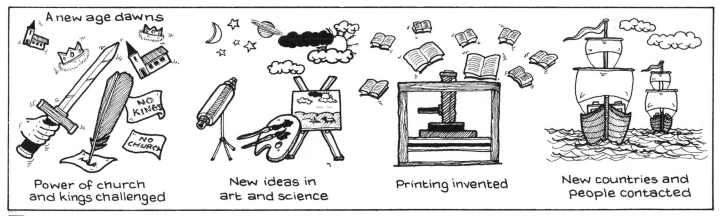
A new age dawns

Power of church and kings challenged

New ideas in art and science

Printing invented

New countries and people contacted

C Summary diagram of the Renaissance way of life.

Questions

1 Look at picture **A**. List the things in the picture which show that the men were interested in science and art.
2 Why would the invention of printing be good for medicine?
3 Look at picture **B**. Why might art like this be good for medicine?
4 What evidence can you find in this chapter to show that the Renaissance was a period of discovery and new ideas? Make a list.

5 Pictures from the Renaissance look very different from those of the Middle Ages. Compare picture **A** with any picture from the Middle Ages (e.g. page 22 or 24). What is different about
a what they show,
b how the pictures are painted, and
c why the pictures are painted?
6 The pictures from the Renaissance seem to be more lifelike than those from the Middle Ages. Does this mean that they are more useful to the historian as evidence about those times? Explain your answer.
7 Why do historians find it difficult to agree about when periods like the Renaissance begin and end?

The Renaissance - medicine

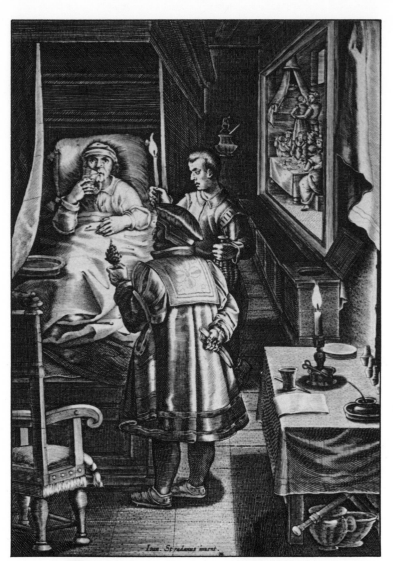

A 17th century doctor visiting a patient. The doctor is shown on the right with his back to us.

B Extract from Henri and Barbara van de Zee's biography of William III (Macmillan, 1973).

"

Since November the previous year (1700) the doctors in England had tried everything possible to get down the . . . swelling: frictions with elderflower water; 'spaw-water', pills made of extract of gentian and lesser centary, powder of crabs' claw, huge pills made of salt of wormwood, crabs' eyes, tartar vitviolate, steel prepared with sulphur. They fed him Epsom salt in chicken broth, purged him with rosin of jalap and extract of rhubarb, and dosed him with tincture of steel . . . his legs remained as swollen as ever and his cough got worse.

"

The biographers go on to say that William's doctors had given him a thorough examination, writing down their findings and the treatments they had prescribed for him. The doctors described the problem as 'a soft pale swelling that retains pits after being pressed with one's finger'. They had once suggested that his legs be tightly bandaged, but he only got worse. Next they tried massage and more pills and purging. All that happened was that William lost his appetite.

William went to Holland soon afterwards and saw some Dutch doctors who totally changed his treatment. They suggested herbal wine, and told him to eat less fruit. William's favourite doctor had a little stove specially made. It was a box made of oak big enough so that the King could sit with his legs and thighs inside it. It was lined with flannel, and on either side burned little lamps filled with spirits of lavender – a smell William liked. It worked wonders; William was delighted with it, but he wasn't a good patient and he soon didn't bother with it, so his condition got worse.

Although his swollen legs caused William lots of pain and discomfort, they were not so serious that they would cause his death. However, along with some of the treatment he was given, they did weaken him considerably. So when, in February 1702, William fell from his horse and broke his collar bone, it did not mend properly and became infected. His doctors tried all the remedies they had suggested earlier but William grew tired of their concoctions and said: 'Believe me, gentlemen, I know particularly well that forced feeding does me no good.' He was right. Within two days he was dead.

You may have noticed that the Renaissance is supposed to have been the period when the ideas of the Greeks and Romans were rediscovered and helped to change the way people thought about the world. However, does this apply to medicine? We have seen that the ideas of Galen and Hippocrates had been studied in parts of the Middle East, Africa and Europe for 1500 years.

Look at the pictures and read about the way in which King William III of England was treated for swollen legs by his doctors. Then make up your mind about whether the Renaissance really did bring about as many changes in medicine as it did in other things – such as science and art.

Questions

1 Read the information about William III. Copy out these sentences, and say if they are true or false. You must give reasons and copy out parts of the chapter to back up your answer.
   a The doctors did not try to find out what was wrong with William.
   b Nothing done by William's doctors helped him.
   c William was a good patient.
2 Explain why the doctors might disagree with each other about the way to treat William.
3 How hygienic were conditions in the room shown in picture A? Mention things seen in the picture to support your answer.

4 Compare picture A with the picture of the medieval doctor (page 24).
   a What similarities and differences do you notice in the treatment of the sick?
   b Do these two pictures prove that the artists' ideas changed between medieval and Renaissance times? Explain your answer.
5 Compare the remedies used to treat William III with those used in the Middle Ages (pages 24-25). How similar are they?
6 How much change had there been in the methods used by doctors compared with those used by Medieval doctors? Explain your answer by comparing picture C with the medieval picture E (page 24).

C A 16th century doctor at work.

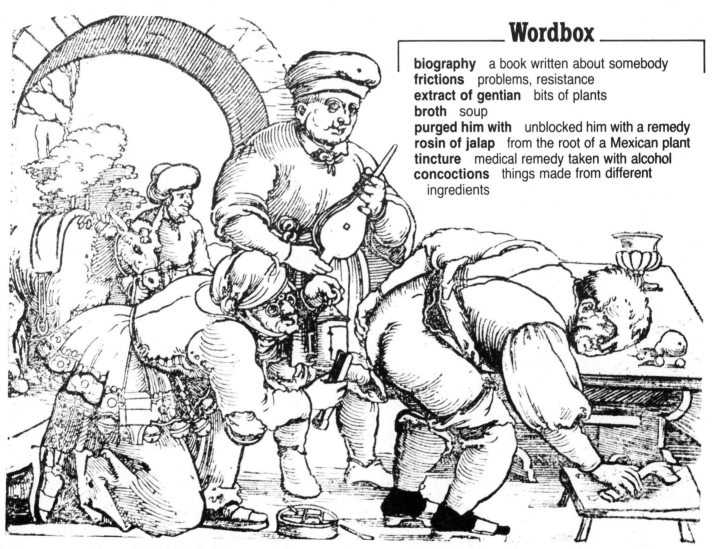

Wordbox

biography a book written about somebody
frictions problems, resistance
extract of gentian bits of plants
broth soup
purged him with unblocked him with a remedy
rosin of jalap from the root of a Mexican plant
tincture medical remedy taken with alcohol
concoctions things made from different ingredients

The modern world - the way of life

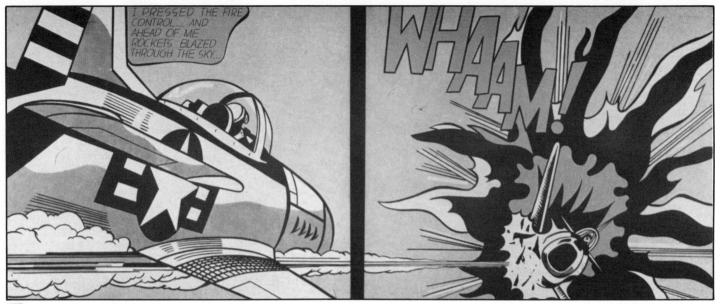

A Whaam! A piece of modern art from Roy Lichtenstein (died 1963).

Government

Although what we have called the 'modern' world is not one of the longest periods in history, it is certainly the one in which most changes have taken place. Governments, along with everything else, have undergone all kinds of alterations. In Europe, the power of royal families has been reduced. Elected parliaments increasingly control the running of countries. At first only a few wealthy people were allowed to vote, but after a good deal of effort most men and women, however poor, became voters.

Democracy, as this system of government is called, is only one of many ways to run a country. In eastern Europe they have a system called communism. Communist countries are controlled by members of the Communist Party, whose stated intention is to run the country for the benefit of all the people in it.

Economy

The change from farming to industry, which has affected many people in modern times, is seen by historians as one of the most important ever. The growth of industry brought about many other changes, particularly in Europe and America. Instead of working in the fields, people worked in factories at machines; they created large industrial cities and a demand for all kinds of goods and services. Today, most of the things around us – including buildings and food – were made in factories of some kind.

These changes to the economies of nations brought power and wealth to a few people and a slow improvement in standards of living for many others.

Industrialization did not affect all the world at the same time. Farming is still the main way to earn a living for many South American, African and Asian peoples.

Technology

To list all the things invented during this period would take up most of this book! Tremendous advances were made in industry, transportation, communication, sources of power, building, farming and everyday life. These developments affected lives throughout the world and have made Europe, America and Japan very rich. However, they have left some countries with few benefits.

Thinking

As scientific knowledge has improved, so the mysteries of the world have been reduced. However, there is not just one set of scientific answers to explain everything. Scientists often argue about how and why things work. It's not just scientists that argue; in fact, if you take any group of people you will find that they disagree about all kinds of things and have plenty of ideas about how the world could be changed for the better. Some would say that if people didn't argue there would be no progress at all. The only trouble is that sometimes people have come to very different conclusions about what things are important for mankind. So although there are many signs of world co-operation in the 20th century, there are also times when people disagree so completely that it leads to demonstrations, riots and even war. There is also another price to pay for progress. Pollution, waste and man-made destruction endanger the lives of many creatures and plants on this planet, including humans! Never in the history of the world has it been possible to destroy so much so quickly.

Wordbox

alterations   changes
government   control of a country
democracy   all the people vote for a
   government
communism   everyone is supposed to be equal
industrialization   development of machinery
   and factories
pollution   harmful waste that affects the
   environment

B Summary diagram of the modern way of life.

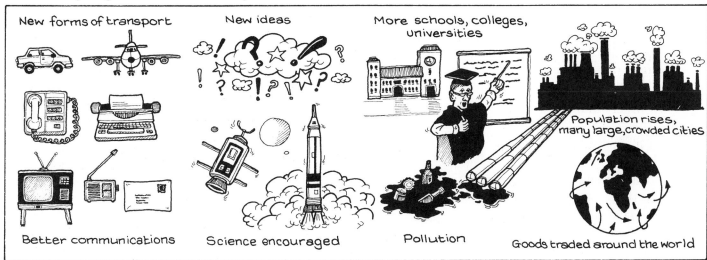

New forms of transport

New ideas

More schools, colleges, universities

Better communications

Science encouraged

Pollution

Population rises, many large, crowded cities

Goods traded around the world

Questions

1 Make a list of some of the things invented or developed during your lifetime. Explain how they have changed people's lives.

2 Compare picture **A** with the Renaissance painting on page 26. What similarities and differences do you notice between the ways the pictures have been painted and the things shown in them?

3 From what you know about the modern way of life, how much change would you have expected to take place in medicine this century. Explain your answers.

The modern world - medicine

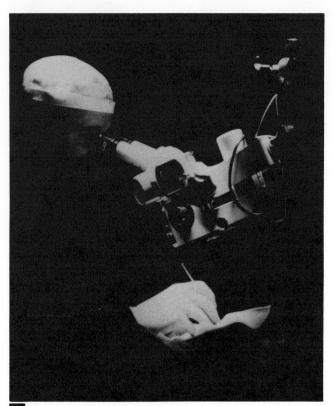

A A micro-surgeon at work.

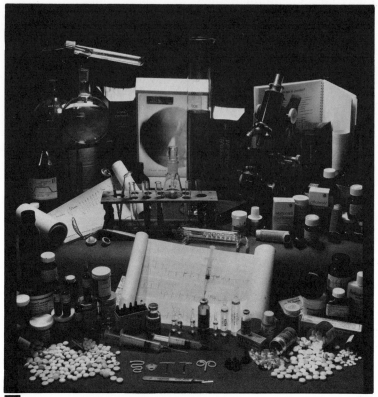

B Modern medical equipment.

Medicine in the 19th and 20th centuries
Most of the important advances made during this period are to be found elsewhere in this book. To find out about these developments, turn to the following pages:

Surgery and the work of Sir James Simpson 1847 (page 39), and Joseph Lister 1865 (page 40).

Public health and Edwin Chadwick 1848 (page 88).

Anatomy and X-rays (page 64).

Causes and cures for illness, see Louis Pasteur 1864 (page 49), Koch 1882 (page 88) and Alexander Fleming 1928 (page 110).

Nursing and the work of Florence Nightingale 1856 (page 78).

As the 19th and 20th centuries progressed, so the health of people living in Europe improved. People lived longer, ate better, grew taller and received better medical care than ever before. There are now only a few diseases that cannot be cured, and for those that cannot, such as Parkinson's disease or AIDS, large amounts of money are being spent on the best facilities to try to find a cure.

There are now huge factories mass producing a wide range of drugs and medical equipment. Millions of pounds can be made from the development and sale of new medicines. There have been some drugs that were not properly tested, resulting in unpleasant side effects. To avoid this, governments now enforce strict rules about how drugs should be tested.

Of all recent developments perhaps the transplanting of human organs is the most remarkable. The work was pioneered by Doctor Christian Barnard of South Africa. In 1967 he performed the first heart transplant operation. Since that time great advances have been made in this type of surgery and now almost any organ can be transplanted. It is also possible to make plastic hearts and fit them inside people. Less drastic, but equally impressive, is the heart pacemaker which can stimulate a weak heart by electrical impulses. The idea was first thought of by a British surgeon W H Walshe in 1863, but it was not until the 1930s that a working model was produced; it weighed 7.2 kilos. Today, pacemakers are small enough to fit inside the body and don't need to be replaced for 10 years. Picture **C** gives you some idea of the range and variety of things that can be done to relieve pain and suffering.

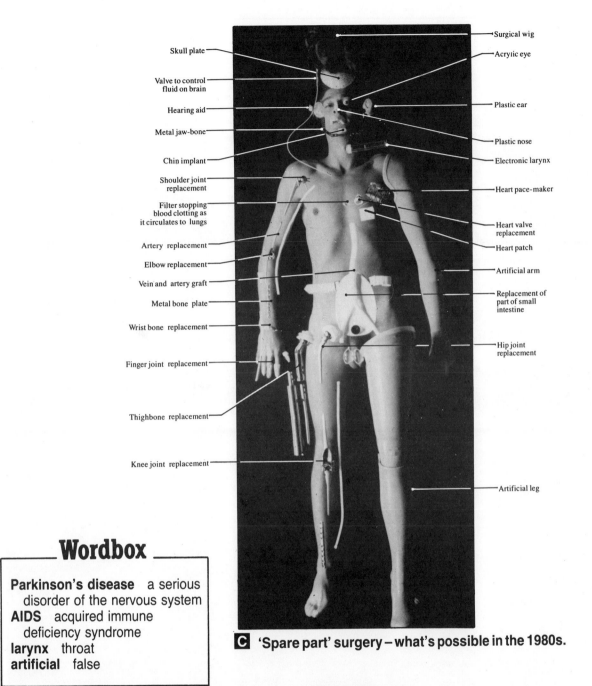

Skull plate

Valve to control
fluid on brain

Hearing aid

Metal jaw-bone

Chin implant

Shoulder joint
replacement

Filter stopping
blood clotting as
it circulates to lungs

Artery replacement

Elbow replacement

Vein and artery graft

Metal bone plate

Wrist bone replacement

Finger joint replacement

Thighbone replacement

Knee joint replacement

Surgical wig

Acrylic eye

Plastic ear

Plastic nose

Electronic larynx

Heart pace-maker

Heart valve
replacement

Heart patch

Artificial arm

Replacement of
part of small
intestine

Hip joint
replacement

Artificial leg

C 'Spare part' surgery – what's possible in the 1980s.

Wordbox

Parkinson's disease a serious
disorder of the nervous system
AIDS acquired immune
deficiency syndrome
larynx throat
artificial false

Questions

1 How does a microscope like the one shown in picture **A** help surgeons?
2 Compare picture **B** with picture **E** (page 24). What similarities and differences are there between modern and medieval equipment?
3 There is now a wide variety of machines used in medicine. Name some *not* mentioned in this chapter and explain their use.
4 Why couldn't the heart pacemaker be developed for use in 1863?

Early forms of surgery : 1

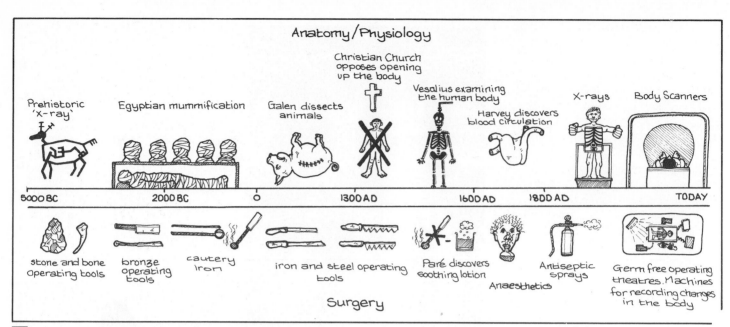

A Diagram showing some changes in human understanding of anatomy, physiology and surgery.

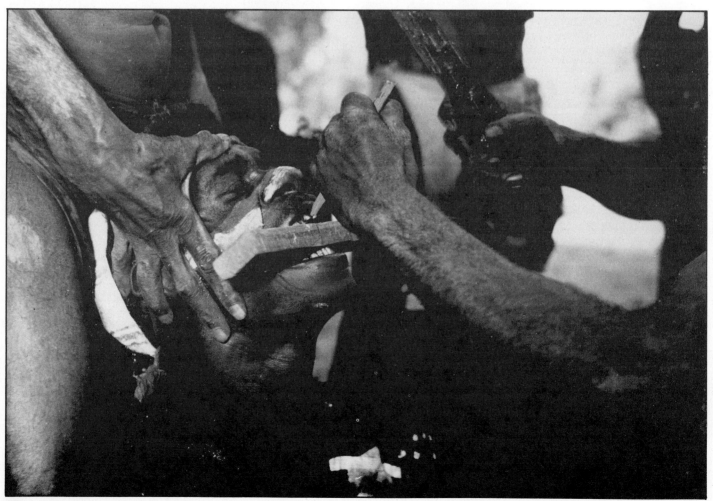

B Aborigine dental operation.

How much progress has there been in surgery? To answer this question we need to know about the body (anatomy) and how it works (physiology).

The next four units are all on the topic of surgery. Later on there is information about anatomy and physiology. Diagram A shows some of the main changes which took place in knowledge about anatomy, physiology and surgery.

When looking at the evidence in the next units, think about these points:

(a) what changes took place,
(b) during which period did the least change take place and why,
(c) during which period did the most change take place and why,
(d) and were some changes more important than others in bringing about change?

How much progress had there been in surgery by the end of the Middle Ages? We can answer this question by studying the evidence left behind from different periods in history.

Prehistoric surgery
When we looked at the chapter on prehistoric societies we saw that holes in skulls provided clues that an operation, called trepanning, had taken place. Perhaps the aim of this operation was to release evil spirits thought to be inside the head. Difficult though it may be to believe, this operation was sometimes carried out successfully; but it must have been painful! We learned more about prehistoric medicine by studying the customs of the Australian aborigines, and if we look at evidence like that shown in photograph **B** we may be able to work out a little more about prehistoric surgery.

Roman and Greek surgery
Simple surgical tools have been found in Roman cities. The Greek doctor, Galen, looked after gladiators as well as emperors and is known to have carried out operations. The ideas of Greek physicians were used by the Romans to protect their soldiers. To conquer and control its mighty empire, Rome needed a fit and healthy army. Military doctors called 'medici' followed the army and carried out operations on the battlefield, like the one seen on this page.

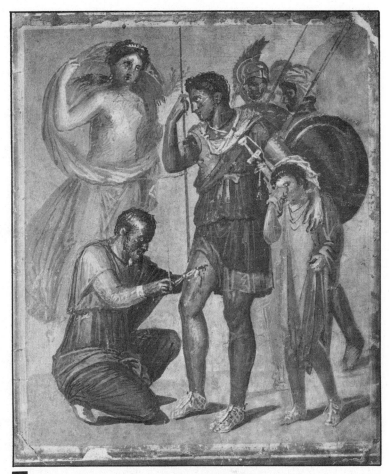

C Painting found on a wall in the Roman city of Pompeii, showing the Roman hero, Aeneas, being treated for a wound on the battlefield.

Questions

Don't do these questions, which refer to diagram **A**, until you thoroughly understand the ideas about surgery described in the next four units.

1 Name one period in which change took place only slowly.
2 Name one period in which change took place quickly.
3 The diagram is not complete; it only shows some of the changes in surgery. Suggest other things or people which might go on the diagram.
4 Diagram **A** might suggest that things got better and medicine developed steadily through time. Do you agree? Explain your answer.

Early forms of surgery : 2

Medieval surgery

Some of the scientific ideas of the Greeks were ignored, forgotten or 'lost' after the fall of the Roman empire. However, Arab doctors had studied Greek books which had been translated into Arabic. They wrote their own books on surgery and these were used by a number of medieval surgeons. They copied the Arab idea of stopping the flow of blood by the use of a cautery iron. A man heated up the fire so that a red-hot iron could 'scorch' the hole in the man's head. No anaesthetic would have been used!

There were two kinds of surgeon in the Middle Ages – the surgeon and the barber surgeon. The surgeons were sometimes educated and wealthy. The barber surgeons were less educated and less wealthy. They did haircutting, tooth pulling, blood letting and a lot of rather unusual jobs – as picture **A** suggests.

Being a medieval surgeon wasn't everybody's idea of a good job! In 1337 a surgeon was thrown into the River Oder because he failed to cure King John of Bohemia of blindness. Pope John XII burned an unsuccessful surgeon. Opposition to surgery was so strong that the school at Montpellier in France closed down its classes in surgery and ordered that none of its students should study or practise surgery. One mdeieval surgeon was advised to 'avoid a bad reputation, because the people, since ancient times, think all surgeons are thieves, man-killers and the worst kind of cheats.' Picture **A** gives us clues about medieval operations.

Renaissance surgery – the work of Ambroise Paré

Ambroise Paré (1510–1590) was a French army surgeon who gained a lot of experience treating soldiers involved in the many wars of that time. He saw the cruelty of war, the suffering of the injured, the low ability of many of the surgeons and the pain inflicted on soldiers who suffered amputations like that seen in picture **B**. Many soldiers bled to death unless their gunshot wounds were scorched with boiling oil or a hot iron. Many must have died from the shock of the cautery iron which had been used to stop their bleeding.

Parés great discovery

One day Paré had treated so many soldiers for gunshot wounds that he ran out of boiling oil. So he tried out a new method of treating the soldiers. He made up a lotion from egg yolk, turpentine and oil of roses, and bathed the wound with the

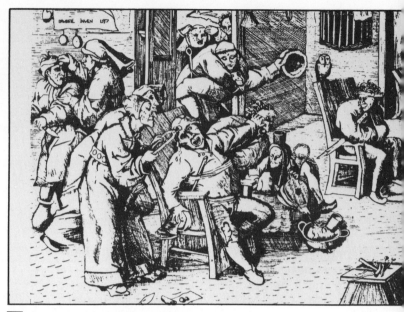

A A medieval barber surgeon.

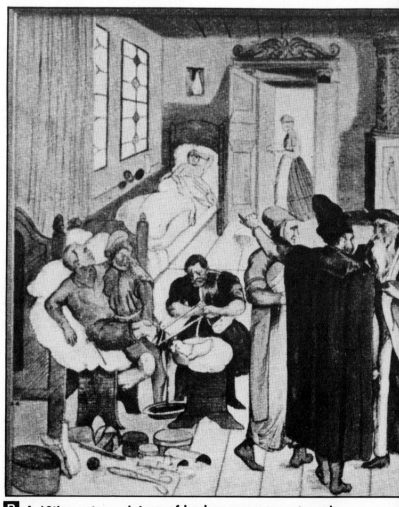

B A 16th-century picture of barber surgeons at work.

lotion. That night he couldn't sleep, terrified by the fear that the men treated by the new lotion would be dead. To his great joy he found that they had survived, and from that day onwards he made up his mind never again to use the cruel method of cautery, but to treat his patients in this new, more humane way. He found that the bleeding could be stopped by using a ligature. This meant tying up the arteries, then bandaging the wound. This method is still used today and has saved countless lives.

Paré wrote down his ideas in a book about surgery *'The Collected Works of Surgery' (1575)*.

C Paré's description of an operation on the Marquis d'Arnet.

"

I found him in high fever, with a yellowish face, the whole body wasted, as of a man very near death. I found his thigh much inflamed, discharging a greenish and very offensive liquid. I found a large cavity in the middle of the thigh. There was a large bed-sore; he could rest neither day nor night. I began to say to the surgeons that I was astonished that they had not made incisions [cuts] in the patient's thigh. They answered me, never would he agree to it; indeed it was near two months since they had been able to get permission to put clean sheets on the bed.

We went back to the patient and I made three openings in his thigh. I got a bed made near his old one, with clean sheets on it; then a strong man put him onto it, and he was thankful to be taken out of his foul stinking bed. Soon after, he asked to sleep, which he did for nearly four hours – and everybody in the house began to rejoice.

"

Paré also produced detailed drawings of new surgical tools, and even made artificial limbs. Although he didn't know much about germs or anaesthetics, he had certainly made improvements in surgery. However, many of his ideas were ignored, and surgeons continued to use the cautery iron and work in terribly filthy conditions. Three hundred years after Paré we find this suggestion written into the visitors' book of an English hospital: 'There should be a positive order that sheets should be changed in ordinary cases at least once a month.'

Much remained to be done – as this quote from a book on the history of medicine suggests: 'After Paré's time, infection in surgery was more frequent than it had been when the cautery was used. The full benefit of the ligature (tying) in controlling bleeding was not obtained until after Lister had shown how surgical infection was spread.'

Wordbox

ligature	something tied tightly

Questions

Use pages 34-37 to study how surgery has changed over the years. Think about whether improvements in surgery came about quickly or slowly, and why. Write your answers on to a chart like the one shown below.

Leave plenty of space between the questions and use a double page so that you have room to explain your ideas.

Questions	Prehistoric	Roman	Medieval	Renaissance
a Where does an operation take place?				
b How is the patient kept still?				
c What tools and equipment are used?				
d What is done to stop pain?				
e What is done to stop bleeding?				
f What is done to stop infection?				

The discovery of anaesthetics

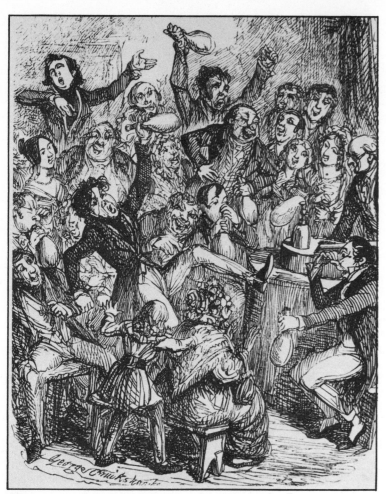

B Cartoon of 1834 by George Cruikshank, showing the audience at a lecture enjoying the effects of laughing gas. This was used as an anaesthetic in early experiments.

anaesthetics had been discovered. There was quite a difference!.

A The operation before and after the use of anaesthetics, as described by Hayden.

"

. . . the patient is brought into the operating theatre, which is crowded with men who are anxious to see the shedding of her blood. She is laid upon the table. She knows the intense agony which she is about to suffer. She is cheered by kind words and the knowledge that it will soon be over and she will be freed forever from the suffering she is going through. She is told to be calm and to keep quiet and still. Assistants hold her struggling body down and the operation begins.

At last it is over. Collapsed with pain, weak from her efforts to break free and bruised from the violence used against her, the girl is carried from the operating theatre to her bed in the wards to recover slowly from the shock.

How would the same case be now?

The patient is lying down, relaxed. She does not need to be surrounded by strong men to force her to keep still or guard against unexpected accidents. The only people needed are the surgeon and his two assistants (to pass him the necessary surgical tools or to help in staunching the flow of blood). The surgeon is not hurried by the demands of pain to complete the operation as soon as possible. He can take his time and coolly go about his work, varying it to suit the needs of the operation and making full use of these benefits.

When the operation is finished, the patient is awakened from her sleep and hears the good news that it is over. The grateful look which answers this news can have no value placed upon it. It is worth a lifetime of effort and trouble.

"

Humphrey Davy, the inventor of a safety lamp for miners, carried out experiments using gas. In 1799 he discovered that if he breathed in nitrous oxide gas it sometimes had strange effects. One day he had a toothache: 'I felt great pain and my gums swelled up badly. On the day that the swelling was at its worst, I breathed three large doses of nitrous oxide. I felt less pain.' This led him on to a very important conclusion: 'As nitrous oxide appears capable of destroying physical pain, it may probably be used during surgical operations.'

Before anaesthetics were used, operations must have been terrible for the patients. We know this because in 1896 a surgeon called Hayden wrote a book in which he described two operations, one of which took place before the introduction of anaesthetics, the other carried out after

In the middle of the 19th century, a number of surgeons were looking for a safe, reliable and successful way of anaesthetizing a patient for the operation. In 1844 Horace Wells used nitrous oxide to remove a tooth. Dr James Simpson, Professor of Midwifery at Glasgow University, had tried using ether to help his patients suffer less pain during childbirth. He found that ether had a nasty smell and didn't always work very well. He thought that something else might be more successful, so he tried out a number of chemicals, one of which was chloroform. He carried out a very unusual experiment, which was to be of great help for millions of patients in the future, but which had a sensational result! One day in 1847, Simpson and two other surgeons, called Keith and Duncan, met in the dining room of Simpson's house. Each man had a glass full of chloroform in front of him. They sniffed the chloroform and began talking and laughing. Then suddenly, they all collapsed and fell on the floor. Fortunately, they all eventually woke up. They had discovered an effective anaesthetic.

Simpson then tried out the chloroform on one of his patients – a woman who was very worried about the pain she would have to go through in childbirth.

However, there was great opposition to anaesthetics at the time of these discoveries. Much of the criticism of Simpson's use of chloroform anaesthetic came from the church. It was thought that it was against God's law to try to stop pain in childbirth. A clergyman wrote: 'Chloroform is a trick of the devil, seeming to help women, but in the end it will rob God of the deep cries which arise in time of trouble for help.' He backed up his idea with a quotation from the Bible: 'Unto the woman, he said, I will greatly multiply thy sorrow; in sorrow shalt thou bring forth children.'

Also causing criticism was the fact that, in the early days, anaesthetics were not always used properly. Some patients still died and there were many accidents.

However, when chloroform was safely and successfully used as an anaesthetic at the birth of Queen Victoria's son, Leopold, a lot of the criticism of Simpson's anaesthetics stopped.

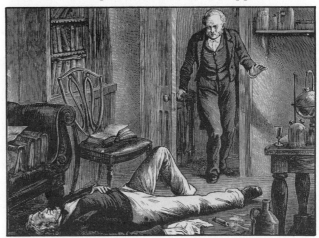

C Simpson's discovery of the effects of chloroform; a drawing depicting the scene when he is discovered by his butler.

Wordbox

anaesthetic   something which removes feeling in order to prevent pain
chloroform   liquid anaesthetic
nitrous oxide   an anaesthetic gas
midwifery   the care of pregnant women

Questions

1 **a** Describe carefully what is happening in the operation shown on the front cover of this book.
   b Compare the front cover with the picture of the medieval amputation (page 36). Does much progress seem to have been made in surgery in the 200 years between the times at which these pictures were drawn? Explain your answer.
2 Read document **A**. List the ways in which anaesthetics improve operations.
3 How did these things affect the story of anaesthetics? Copy out the list of reasons, or factors and explain how each of them played a part in the story.
   a *Communications:* Many surgeons and scientists were experimenting with chemicals and wanted to exchange ideas across Europe.
   b *Science:* Different types of experiments were tried in the 19th century.
   c *Chance:* See picture **C**.
   d *Economy:* The industrial revolution led to a demand by factory owners for knowledge about chemicals, gases etc.
4 What does cartoon **B** show and what point do you think the person who drew the cartoon was trying to make about the use of laughing gas as an anaesthetic?
5 What happened in James Simpson's experiment and what do you think it tells us about the sort of person he was?
6 If anaesthetics were such a good idea, why do you think so many people were opposed to them? Explain your answer carefully.
7 How important do you think the discovery of anaesthetics was in the history of medicine? Give reasons for your answer.

Joseph Lister and modern surgery

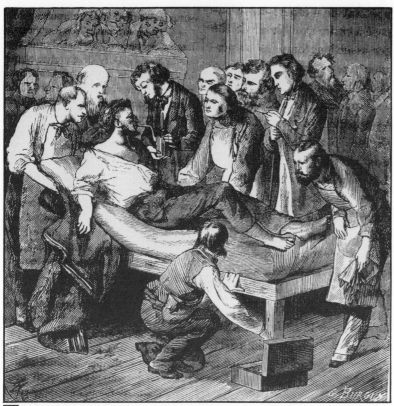

A William Morton (1819–1868) demonstrating the safety of ether at Massachusetts Hospital, USA, 1846.

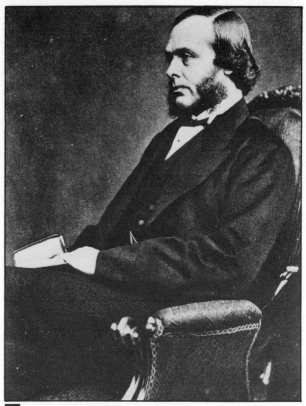

B Joseph Lister (1827–1912).

Anaesthetics meant that longer, more difficult operations could be done with less pain for the patients. However, there was still a lot that needed to be done before surgical operations could be carried out more safely.

Many patients were still dying of blood poisoning or infection after an operation. Even though Louis Pasteur had published his theory that germs cause disease, many doctors didn't believe him. Because they didn't know what caused disease, they didn't understand how important it was to be clean both in the operating theatre and in the hospital ward. Doctors rarely washed their surgical coats and operated on their patients wearing clothes that were stained with blood and pus. The dirtier the coat, the better the surgeon, many people thought at the time!

However, these ideas eventually changed. Photograph **C** shows a 'modern' operation. You can see that there have been some important changes in people's ideas about surgery. The man who has been given the praise for bringing in many of these new ideas was called Joseph Lister. He was born in 1827 and studied medicine in London, Edinburgh and at several important hospitals in Europe. He became a professor at Glasgow University.

One day Lister read an article in a scientific paper. It had been written by Louis Pasteur and described his theory that germs cause disease. Leading scientists all over Europe could find out quickly about each other's ideas by reading these scientific papers and attending international conferences. Lister took Pasteur's idea and applied it to surgery. Suddenly it seemed obvious why so many patients were dying in hospital. The surgeons were not taking care to prevent the spread of infections and illness through germs.

Lister insisted that the operating theatre, the surgeon, his clothes and equipment were kept clean. Today, all surgeons scrub their hands very carefully and go through a 'clean barrier' before beginning any operation. However, Lister knew that it was not enough just to keep clean. He also had to find something that would kill the germs and stop infection.

Wordbox

gangrene a serious illness when parts of the body, because of infection, start to decay

40

The carbolic spray

Lister decided to use a carbolic spray to clean both the wounds and the surgical tools. He had read that carbolic acid had been used to help treat the sewage in the big industrial cities. If it was strong enough to treat sewage, perhaps it would be powerful enough to kill germs.

Lister tried out his idea in a daring experiment. An 11-year-old boy called James had been run over by a cart. His leg had been broken. In the old days a surgeon might have cut off the leg, to save the boy from gangrene. However, Lister decided to treat the wound with the spray and then to put splints on the leg. For days Lister waited to see if infection would set in. To his great delight and relief Lister found that the bone had healed up and the boy was not going to die of infection.

Lister was made a lord towards the end of his life, and a statue was put up of him. He is thought to have been so important that surgery is now divided into two periods of time – *before* Lister and *after* Lister. When he died in 1912 the Royal College of Surgeons paid this tribute to Lister: 'His work will last for all time. Humanity will bless him evermore and his fame will be immortal.'

With less risk of infection and, under improved anaesthetics, more complex internal operations were possible. But there were still difficulties after Lister, one of them being how to stop bleeding. Progress had been made but there was still a long way to go.

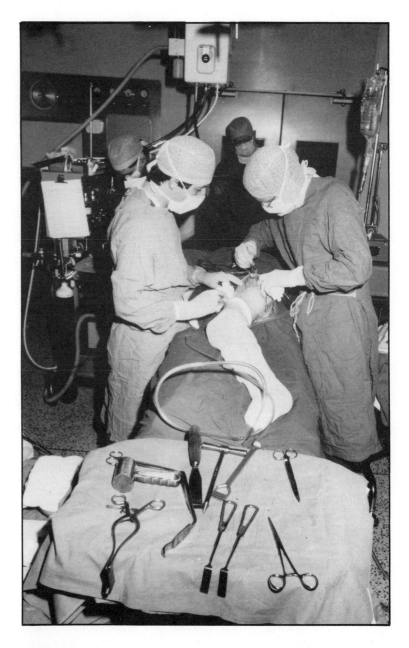

C *(Right)* **A modern operating theatre.**

Questions

1 Look at print **A**. How safe do you think the operation was for the patient? Back up your answer by mentioning things in the picture.

2 Compare pictures **A** and **C**. Make a list of ways surgery has improved since the first operation with anaesthetic.

3 How important do you think the following things were in helping Lister:
  a good communications (e.g. scientific papers), and
  b industry (carbolic acid)?

4 How big do you think the change that Lister made to surgery was? Explain your answer and back it up by copying at least two sentences from the chapter.

5 Use the information from this chapter to fill in a final column of the 'surgery through the ages' chart (see page 37). Give this column the title 'Modern operations – after Lister'.

Explaining sickness

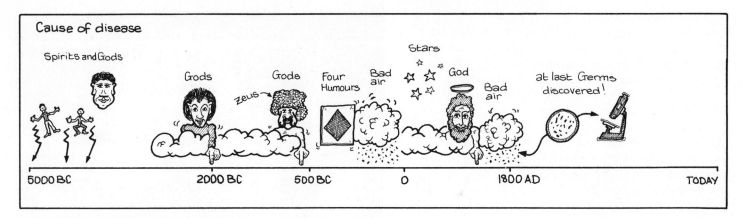

Cause of disease

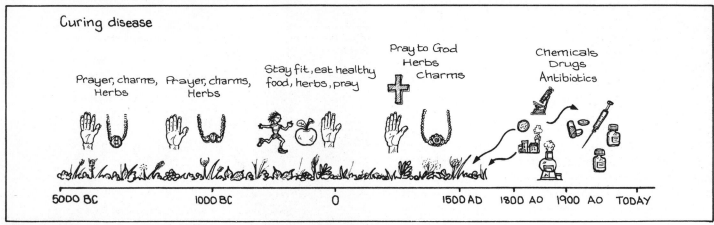

Curing disease

A Diagram showing causes and cures of diseases throughout the ages.

Diagram **A** shows some of the main changes which took place in knowledge about the cause and cure of disease. When looking at the evidence of the next seven units, think about these points:

(a) what changes took place,
(b) during which period did most change take place,
(c) during which period did least change take place,
(d) which ideas were more important than others in bringing about or holding back change?

Before the cause of disease was discovered, it made perfectly good sense to many groups of people to believe that illness, like everything else in the world, was the work of the gods. This idea can be found in many religions and has lasted for thousands of years.

The Egyptians, for example, worshipped Imhotep as a healing god. He was probably a successful physician to a pharaoh, who long after his death was treated as a god. Statues to Imhotep have been found in the homes of ancient Egyptians.

Gods like Bes and Sekhmet were said to scare away disease in Egypt. The Greeks also had a healing god, Asklepios, and temples dedicated to Asklepios have been found all over Greece.

The Holy Bible told Christians about the power of God:

B An extract from the Epistle of James in the New Testament.

"

Is any sick among you? Let him call for the elders of the church. Let them pray for him, anointing him with oil in the name of the Lord. And the prayer of faith shall save the sick, and the Lord shall raise him up.

"

The power of God was on many people's minds in times of plague – as the plague pamphlet of 1665 suggests (picture **C**).

Just as in the world today, people in the 17th century also thought that God passed on his healing power through some humans.

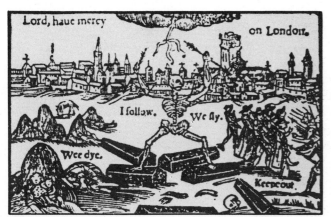

C Pamphlet from a time of plague in London, 1665.

D 'Several Surgical Treaties' by the leading English surgeon, Richard Wiseman, 1676 (during the reign of Charles II).

"

Diseases such as scrofula can be cured if His Majesty touches the patient. It is not the air, nor the journey, nor the imagination nor the token hung around the neck that brings about the cure. It is the holy power of healing given to the sovereign which is the cure. I have seen His Majesty make numerous cures. The gift was given to the Kings of England by Almighty God. The leper: 'Lord, if you will, you can make me clean.' And he put forward his hand and touched him saying: 'I will be clean.' And immediately the leprosy left him.

"

Apart from the powers of gods, people through the ages have thought that the stars were important in causing and curing sickness.

E Statement by the surgeon Guy de Chauliac at the time of the Black Death (1348).

"

The cause of the plague can be found in the position of the planets, Saturn, Jupiter and Mars in the sign of Aquarius.

"

Wordbox

pestilence disease
atmospheric to do with air

F From 'The Black Death', edited by J Nohl, 1971.

"

Comets were blamed for all great plagues. The Roman writer Seneca declared comets to be evil things which appeared before disease, war and earthquakes. Hippocrates, the Greek, taught that 'Comets and eclipses of the sun and moon were the cause of pestilences (sicknesses).' Comets were also said to have appeared before the Black Death. From the position of the comet to the other stars and planets could be worked out which country and which people had most to fear from the plague.

"

G From 'Faults of Physicians', by the 13th-century writer Roger Bacon.

"

Physicians do not study the heavenly bodies, on which all things depend. The whole of medical practice is based on the study of atmospheric changes due to the influence of the spheres and the stars. A physician who does not know how to take into account the positions of the planets can do no healing, unless he happens to heal people by chance.

"

Questions

1 What evidence is there in document **D** to suggest that people believed in other cures of disease, besides the power of God, in the 17th century?
2 Read documents **E** to **G**.
   Do you think the belief that the stars caused disease helped medical progress, or held progress back? Explain your answer.

Don't do these questions, about diagram **A**, until you thoroughly understand the ideas about causes and cures described in the next six units.

3 Name one period in which change took place slowly and one quickly.
4 Digram **A** is not complete. It only shows a few of the changes in knowledge about the causes and cures of disease. Suggest other things which might go on the diagram.
5 Diagram **A** might suggest that things got better and medicine developed steadily through time. Do you agree?
6 Does the discovery of germs mean that we understand the cause of all disease? (see page 54).

The four humours

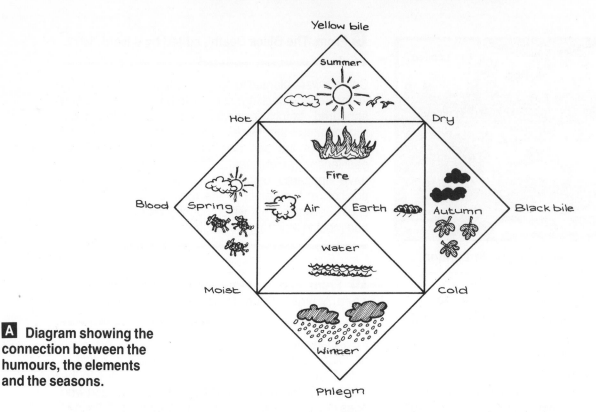

A Diagram showing the connection between the humours, the elements and the seasons.

Greek philosophers came to realize that other explanations were possible for some of the things that people had, in the past, thought of as being the acts of gods or spirits. By careful observation and experiment, they realized that certain things could be predicted (worked out before they happened). A simple example would be the changing seasons of the year.

They went so far as to say that all the things in the world were made up of four basic elements: earth, air, fire and water. Greek doctors, some of whom were philosophers, took this idea a bit further by saying that the human body was made up of these four elements. They didn't mean that the body was actually on fire or contained lumps of earth. No, the body had all these elements, but in the form of liquids. They called them 'humours'. Each humour was connected with an element. The humours were phlegm, blood, yellow bile and black bile. Blood and phlegm were pretty easy to spot; yellow bile and black bile were both supposed to be found deep inside the body.

The Greeks took the idea even further by saying that so long as there were just about equal amounts of these four humours inside the body, then a person would be healthy. But if, for any reason, one particular humour grew larger than the rest and took up more of the body than it should, then there was a very great danger of illness.

The humours got bigger, or smaller, because of the season of the year. Winters were cold and wet, so the humour connected to coldness and wetness, phlegm, increased. If you had too much phlegm in your body, you might suffer from a runny nose or a cold. Spring was moist but warm, so this was connected with blood. If you had too much blood in your body, you might have a nose bleed or dysentery. Summer was hot, and so linked with yellow bile. If you had too much yellow bile in your body you might be feverish, have yellowish skin and vomit. Autumn was cool and linked with black bile. If you had too much black bile in your body, you might have stomach pains and sickness.

Why did the Greeks think like this? They were very good at observing things, they looked closely at what happened to sick people and realized that at certain times of the year some illnesses were more common than others. Coughs and colds were more frequent in the winter for example. So it was not difficult for them to put together their idea about the four elements of the world with the four things they saw when people were ill. This could then be combined with the four seasons, each of which seemed to bring different medical problems.

Phlegm, blood, yellow bile and black bile might have been common signs or symptoms of different illnesses, but they were not the cause of illness.

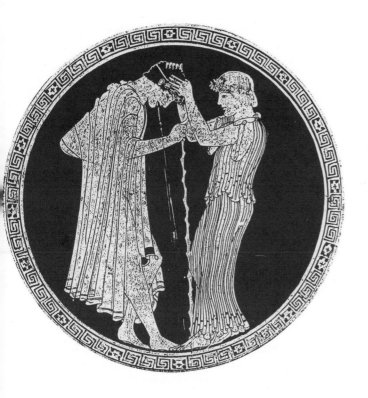

B Picture from a Greek bowl about 480 BC.

C The humours.

Questions

1 Diagram **C** shows the humours in the body. They are out of balance. Copy the chart, showing which is the biggest humour in each season. Shade each humour differently. Also, fill in which illness is connected with each humour. The first one is done for you.
2 Look at picture **B**.
  a Which humour might be out of balance?
  b In what season might this happen?
3 What is the medical word for the signs of illness?
4 Look at diagram **A** . In what ways was the four humours idea wrong as a way of explaining why people got ill?
5 Look back at the section on Explaining Sickness (pages 42-43). Why does the four humours idea seem to be a better way of explaining illness than spirits, gods, or planets?

Wordbox

dysentery	bowel disorder

Key: B = Blood   P = Phlegm   BB = Black Bile   YB = Yellow Bile

	Humour	Season	Illness		Humour	Season	Illness
YB, B, BB, P	Air	Spring	nose bleed	BB			
YB				P			

Edward Jenner and smallpox

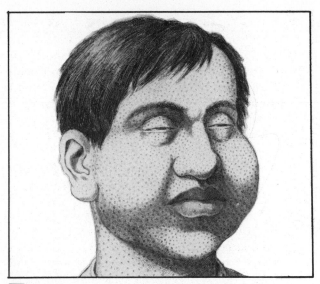

A Smallpox sufferer in the early days after the beginning of the eruption.

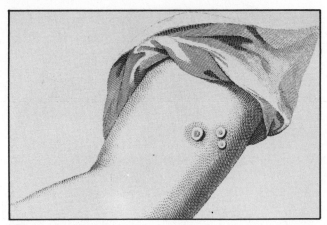

C The arm of Sarah Nelmes, showing the 'pustulous sore', from Jenner's 'Enquiry into the Causes and Effects of the Variolae Vaccinae', 1798.

Infectious diseases have terrified people throughout history. Man often seems powerless to stop them; sometimes they bring death to large numbers of a population. Many writers have described what happens in an epidemic of smallpox. One of these descriptions is in document **B**.

B Part of a description of the death from smallpox of Queen Mary II of England, by the historian Lord Macaulay.

> . . . the plague had been more rapid, but visited our shores only once or twice within living memory; smallpox was always there, filling the churchyards with corpses. It tormented with constant fear all those whom it had not yet hit, leaving on those it did not kill the horrible traces of its power. . .

For hundreds of years there were many country doctors who had spent their lives dealing with smallpox victims. One of them was Edward Jenner (1749–1823). He observed that milkmaids didn't get smallpox. He put forward the idea that perhaps these milkmaids didn't get smallpox because they had got a 'protecting' disease from the cows they worked with. This disease was called cowpox. The signs of this protecting disease were sores on the milkmaids' hands, like the one shown in picture **C**.

Jenner decided to carry out a scientific experiment. He tested out his idea that you could be protected from smallpox if you were infected with cowpox. It was to be a very risky and dangerous experiment – especially when you remember that it took place in the year 1796, which was long before people knew about germs and viruses. It involved a milkmaid called Sarah Nelmes, whose infected hand is shown in the picture above, and a healthy 8-year-old boy.

D Jenner's first vaccination experiment, described in 'Life of Jenner', by Baron, 1838.

> Matter was taken from the hand of Sarah Nelmes, who had been infected by her master's cows, and inserted by two cuts into the arms of James Phipps, a healthy boy of about eight years old. It was necessary to find out if he was safe from smallpox. It was put to the test on July 1st. Variolous matter, taken from a pustule, was carefully inserted – but no disease followed.

The experiment was a complete success. Jenner had discovered the first real vaccination against smallpox. He published his work in 1798, and the government awarded him a grant of £30,000. However, there were many people who were opposed to Jenner's new ideas.

A letter published soon after Jenner's work complained about Jenner's 'unsuccessful experiment' and accused Jenner of producing a vaccine which failed to stop people dying of smallpox. People were slow to accept Jenner's ideas. Almost 70 years after Jenner's experiment, one of his supporters wrote document **E**.

E Description of smallpox by Sir James Simpson, 1864.

"

This terrible disease hits the population all over the island. But if in any one year a catastrophe killed all the people in a county, slaughtered four or five regiments, or wiped out five or six times the numbers of members of the House of Commons, that would terrify the public, and the strongest action would be called for to stop it happening again. I believe that the similar amount of human slaughter caused every year by smallpox is preventable. The hygienic measures needed would be neither difficult nor expensive and would save thousands from death. Why should it be thought harsh or severe that people affected with smallpox should be isolated and prevented from dealing out destruction and death to all they come into contact with.

During the long European wars after the French Revolution 5 or 6 million human lives were lost. In Europe, vaccination has already preserved from death a greater number of human beings than were sacrificed during these wars. Jenner's vaccination had saved far more human lives than the sword of Napoleon destroyed.

England spent millions on these wars and gave titles and pension to the soldiers who were most successful in fighting those battles and destroying their fellow men. Yet Jenner saved 30,000 of her subjects every year.

"

Eventually, governments passed laws which introduced vaccination. Chart **G** shows what happened to the number of people who died from smallpox in Germany after a vaccination law was brought in.

Thanks to modern medicine, the disease smallpox has been almost completely wiped out in many countries of the world.

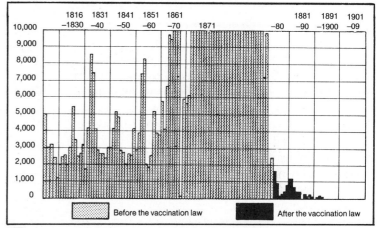

G The effects of the vaccination laws in Germany, 1816–1901.

Wordbox

epidemic a widespread disease
vaccination something given to prevent one getting a disease

Questions

1 **a** What was Jenner's idea about smallpox?
  b How did Jenner prove his idea and why was it so risky?
2 If Jenner wanted to prove that cowpox prevented smallpox, why didn't he just inoculate Sarah Nelmes with smallpox?
3 Was Jenner's discovery just a matter of luck? Give reasons for your answer.
4 The beliefs depicted in cartoon **F** seem ridiculous today, but they were taken seriously in the 19th century. Explain carefully what you think the reasons for this were.
5 Look at chart **G**. Why do you think a vaccination law was introduced in 1873, rather than any other year? Mention things from the chart in your answer.
6 How does picture **A** help us understand the fear of smallpox described in document **B**?

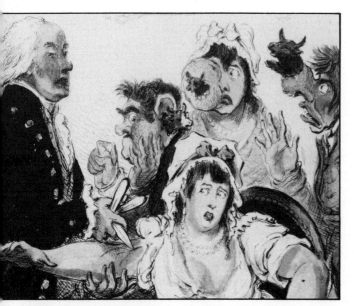

F A cartoon by Gillray in 1802 shows the fears of many people at that time.

The spread of infection

In the past people could not explain the causes of disease in scientific terms. In this section we will examine some of the things which people thought caused diseases like the Black Death. This plague killed about 75 million people in the middle of the 14th century. These documents show how people reacted to it.

A From 'The Black Death', edited by J Nohl, 1971.

"

Many people thought that to get rid of the plague it was necessary to 'break up' the air. Various ways of doing this were tried. Church bells were rung, and muskets were fired. Many people kept canaries in their rooms, to fly about and keep the air moving. It was also thought that speckled spiders, lizards and toads would purify the polluted air and absorb the poison which had been brought by the plague.

Dishes with new milk and small pieces of warm, freshly baked bread were placed in rooms to absorb the poison. Large herds of oxen and cows were driven through towns, to improve the air. The writer, Cardanus, recommended that people live in stables, so that they could get nearer to the breath of horses.

"

B Calendar of Close Rolls (official government document), 1349.

"

To the Lord Mayor of London. Order to cause the human dung and other filth lying in the streets and lanes in the city and its suburbs to be removed with all speed to places far distant . . . and to cause the city and suburbs to be cleaned from all odour so that no greater cause of death may arise from such smells.

The king has learned how the city and suburbs . . . are so foul with the filth from out of the houses by day and night that the air is infected and the city poisoned to the danger of men . . . especially by the contagious sickness which increases daily.

"

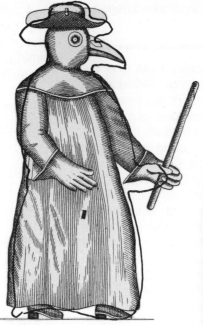

C Plague doctor's outfit in the 18th-century.

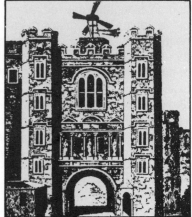

D A windmill put up at Newgate Prison by the Reverend Hales to get rid of the 'bad air' he thought caused disease. It made the prison less smelly.

Questions

1 a Read document **A**. List the cures suggested by those who thought that the air caused the plague.
   b The people who lived in the Middle Ages were not stupid, so why do you think they couldn't work out the real cause of the plague?
2 Explain why it seemed sensible to believe that bad air caused plagues and diseases.
3 Draw the plague doctor's outfit (picture **C**), and explain what it tells us about 18th century ideas about the cause of disease.
4 a Look at picture **D**. How did the Reverend Hales try to treat disease in the prison?
   b 'The Reverend Hales misunderstood the cause of disease, so his cure was bound to be wrong.' Do you agree or disagree with this statement? Explain your answer.
5 According to document **B** why did the king have to order the Lord Mayor to do something about the filth?

Wordbox

odour smell
contagious easily spreading

Louis Pasteur (1822–1895), a Frenchman, made some very important breakthroughs in medicine. He was a teacher at a French university, and worked in a large medical laboratory. He had originally been asked by a wine company to solve a problem. Sometimes wine went bad whilst it was being made. This cost wine companies a lot of money. Pasteur worked away for years and eventually discovered, when he looked closely at bad wine through a microscope, that there were tiny creatures in it. We call these creatures germs. He thought that these might be the cause of the problem.

He had to stop these germs from turning the wine bad. He tried lots of methods, such as adding chemicals, but found that they made the wine taste horrible. In the end he discovered that, by heating up the wine and then cooling it down, the germs were killed off.

Pasteur began to look at other liquids and found germs or microbes in all sorts of things. He was able to make milk much safer by the same method he had used with wine. This process of heating up liquids and cooling them down to kill microbes is called pasteurization. Today some of our milk is named after him.

Germs came from the air, and were not made inside the liquids themselves. He managed to prove this by making up two lots of liquid in which he knew germs would be seen after a few days. One lot he kept sealed up, the other he left in the open air. After a few days he looked at both liquids through a microscope and discovered that the one which had been sealed up had not gone off and had no germs in it. The one left in the open air had gone bad and was full of germs. This proved to Pasteur that germs were carried in the air and did not come from inside things.

Pasteur had found out that microbes lived in many different things. He then thought that microbes might cause diseases, because they obviously turned things bad. He had heard about the work of Edward Jenner (see page 46) who had proved that vaccination could stop smallpox. Jenner couldn't prove what caused diseases like smallpox, but Pasteur thought he could show how Jenner's vaccination idea worked.

When Pasteur examined healthy people's blood he found that there were not many germs in it. But when he examined the blood of people who had terrible diseases he found lots of germs. So Pasteur was able to prove that germs caused disease. He went on to find vaccinations for chicken pox, cholera, diphtheria, anthrax and rabies.

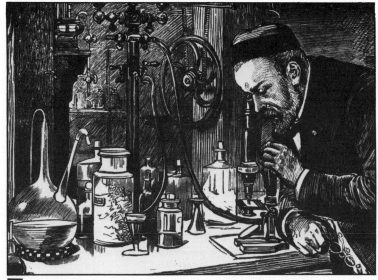

E Louis Pasteur in his laboratory.

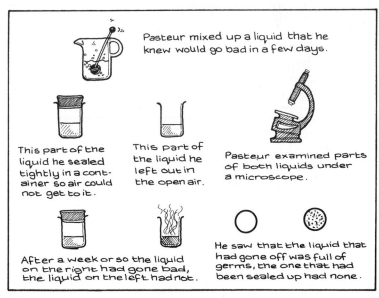

Pasteur mixed up a liquid that he knew would go bad in a few days.

This part of the liquid he sealed tightly in a container so air could not get to it.

This part of the liquid he left out in the open air.

Pasteur examined parts of both liquids under a microscope.

After a week or so the liquid on the right had gone bad, the liquid on the left had not.

He saw that the liquid that had gone off was full of germs, the one that had been sealed up had none.

F Diagram showing Pasteur's experiment.

Questions

1 How could Pasteur prove his idea was true? (Look at diagram F.)
2 Read paragraph 1 on this page. Then read the story of Jenner (page 46). What things made it easy for Pasteur to discover germs, but hard for Jenner?
3 Which industry helped in the discovery of germs, and why?
4 Pasteur's discovery has been described as one of the greatest breakthroughs in medicine. Why do you think it was so important?

The battle against deadly diseases

Once Louis Pasteur had made the all-important discovery that germs cause disease, many other scientists began to copy his ideas and methods. Chart **A** shows some of the other deadly germs which were found in the years following Pasteur's breakthrough.

A Chart showing causes and cures – some important dates.

1883 Cholera germ found
1884 Tetanus identified
1894 Cause of the plague found
1905 Cholera vaccine developed
1906 Vitamins identified
1921 Insulin discovered (it helps cure diabetes)
1928 Fleming discovered penicillin
1935 Gerhardt Domagk developed the sulphonomide prontosil
1942 Penicillin mass produced in the USA
1954 Polio vaccine developed
1965 Measles vaccine developed

Graph **B** shows how quickly the number of people dying from tuberculosis has fallen over the last century.

B Graph showing the fall in annual death rate from tuberculosis in England and Wales, 1834–1960.

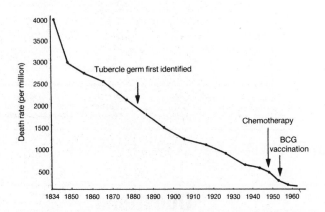

The person who found the bacillus (germ) for tuberculosis was Robert Koch (1843–1910). He came from a poor family in Germany but worked hard enough to qualify as a doctor. He was a very determined, ambitious man and soon became a district medical officer. He went to scientific meetings and read medical papers, so he was able to keep up with the latest ideas of men like Pasteur.

Robert Koch used the scientific methods which had worked so well for Louis Pasteur. The aim was to find the germ which caused a disease, by isolating it. This was done by growing the germ on a single glass plate and studying it carefully with a microscope. Once he had found the cause of the disease, it was possible for other people to find cures for it and to produce vaccines. His methods were copied by some of the other scientists whose discoveries are shown in chart **A**. Some of their names are almost forgotten, but their work is amongst the most important of all that done in the 20th century.

One of those scientists was Paul Ehrlich. He worked with Robert Koch's team in Berlin. Ehrlich was helped by the chemical industry, which was interested in producing coloured dyes. Some doctors realized that this could help medicine, because different coloured dyes could show up different bacteria under the microscope and even kill them.

Ehrlich's team used this method to find ways of killing the deadly germs but leaving the rest of the body safe. The story (document **C**), from Ehrlich's biography, tells us how one of Ehrlich's team found Salversan 606, which had the power to kill the deadly syphilis germ.

The scientist was called Dr Hata, and we join the story at the moment at which he told Ehrlich that 606 could kill the syphilis germ.

C From 'Paul Ehrlich' by Martha Marquandt.

66

Having made his first experiments, Dr Hata came to show Ehrlich his records and said with his usual polite bows, 'Only first trials . . . only preliminary general view. Believe 606 very efficacious. . .'

Ehrlich looked at the records and said, astonished, 'No, surely not? It was all minutely tested by Dr R and he found nothing, nothing. . . More than a year ago we laid aside 606 as being ineffective, worthless. You are sure you are not mistaken, Dr Hata?'

Hata pointed to the records of the experiments and said, shrugging his shoulders, 'I found that, Herr Gheimrat [director].' 'Then it must be repeated, dear Hata, repeated,' said Ehrlich.

. . . One morning he came quickly into his laboratory, followed by Dr Hata. 'Well, my dear Hata, what have you found out now?' asked Ehrlich, coming nearer.

With repeated nods of the head, Hata replied, 'Always 606 is best.' 'Incredible,' said Ehrlich. 'What an incapable good-for-nothing!' he exclaimed, his big eyes looking at Dr Hata over the tops of his spectacles. Hata looked scared and stretched out his arms as if in defence. Ehrlich put his hand on Hata's shoulder, soothingly, and shook his head. 'Oh, not you,' he said, 'not you. No, the other fellow before you.'

Then Dr Hata beamed with delight and grinning broadly he repeated, 'The stupid good-for-nothing!'

"

The battle against disease, and other causes of death, continues. Even though many infectious diseases can be controlled, chart **D** and poster **E** show that other problems face doctors today. As will be seen later in this book, modern medical knowledge is often used to prevent illness rather than just cure it.

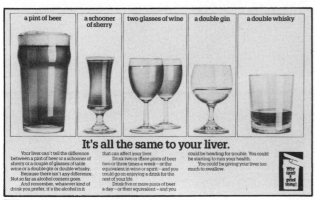

E Health Education Council poster, 1986.

D Chart showing the main causes of death in Britain, 1900–1968. (To the nearest thousand.)

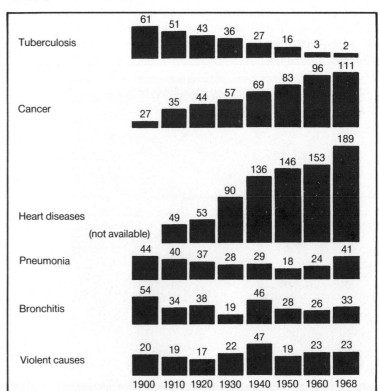

	1900	1910	1920	1930	1940	1950	1960	1968
Tuberculosis	61	51	43	36	27	16	3	2
Cancer	27	35	44	57	69	83	96	111
Heart diseases	(not available)	49	53	90	136	146	153	189
Pneumonia	44	40	37	28	29	18	24	41
Bronchitis	54	34	38	19	46	28	26	33
Violent causes	20	19	17	22	47	19	23	23

Wordbox

isolating separating	**efficacious** works well
viruses germs	**minutely** very carefully
preliminary early	**ineffective** doesn't work

Questions

1 Look at chart **A**. Why was it that the causes of terrible diseases like cholera and the plague should be found within a few years of each other at the end of the 19th century?
2 Look at graph **B**. The death rate from tuberculosis was falling even before the cause of the disease was found. Why may this have been so?
3 Find evidence from these two pages to show how the following factors have affected the fight against disease during the last century:
   a better communications,
   b new technology,
   c the needs of industry, and
   d action taken by governments.
4 Read document **C**. Hata, Ehrlich, Koch and Pasteur all worked in the same sort of way.

Describe how they worked and why this way of working was likely to lead to new discoveries in medicine.
5 Look at chart **D**.
   a Without writing down any figures, how would you describe the change in the types of disease which have killed people in Britain this century?
   b Suggest reasons why the figure for deaths from violent causes was so much higher in 1940 than in any of the other years shown.
6 Why was poster **E** made, and what do you think it tells us about changing attitudes towards death in Britain in recent years?
7 Chart **D** is a table of statistics. What are the advantages and disadvantages of statistics to the medical historian?

A world view

Great technological progress has been made in the 20th century. Medicine is just one of many areas of science that have been affected by changes in technology. Picture **A** shows how a medical problem which had no real cure a few decades ago can now be treated.

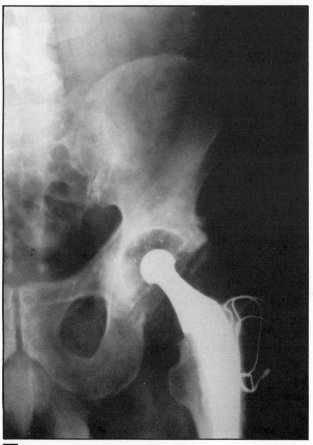

A X-ray picture of an artificial hip.

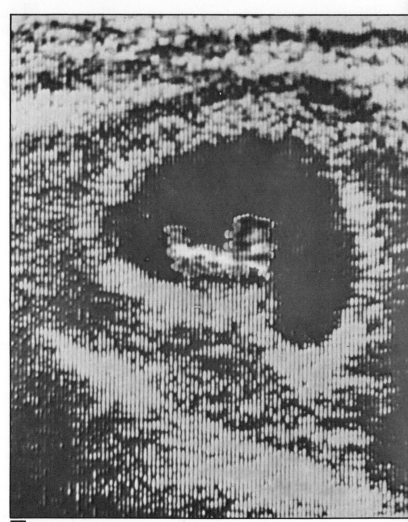

B Ultrasound picture of a child in its mother's womb.

The X-ray in picture **A** shows the head of the thigh bone replaced by a metal ball on a pin which has been put into the bone. The ball fits into a plastic cup which is then glued into the hip-bone socket. The unit on Roentgen (page 64) gives us an idea of how important X-rays have become. Some of the fantastic possibilities in spare-part surgery can be seen on page 33.

New machines are being invented to help the medical profession. Picture **B** is an ultrasound picture of the womb of an expectant mother. Ultrasound pictures are taken by high-pitched sound waves which are passed through the body and are reflected by objects such as muscle or bone. These echoes are made into pictures by computers. Ultrasound can show the age of the baby and its position in the womb.

Scientific medicine has changed our knowledge of the causes and cures of illness, but there are still lots of different ideas about treatments, as we see in document **C**.

C From an article called 'Need your doctor be so useless?' It was written by Dr Andrew Malleson and printed in the 'Observer Review', 14 January, 1973.

"

Need your doctor be so useless?

It would be unjust to suggest that doctors and their treatments never do good. Once it is known exactly what is wrong with the mechanism of our bodies, it is possible to know what, if anything, will put it right. This is the basis of medicine, and it has proved dramatically effective.

It is not treatment that now keeps such large numbers of us alive and well in the West: it is good preventive medicine and improved hygiene that does. By ensuring that sewage is kept out of the water supply, they have abolished typhoid and cholera. By providing vaccination against smallpox, whooping cough, diphtheria, tuberculosis and poliomyelitis, they have almost eliminated these diseases. By adding fluoride to our water supply in those areas where its natural concentration is low, they provide an element which is needed by our children for the growth of decay-resistant teeth. Inspectors from their departments try to ensure that the food we buy is healthy. They enforce the Factory Acts that limit the exposure of workers and miners to harmful substances. How then can our good health be further improved?

The answer is simple, though perhaps discomforting. We can do it ourselves. Ordinary citizens are now in the best position to make effective advances in the prevention of disease. The ball is in our court.

"

We should not think that medical ideas and problems are similar all over the world. Chart **D** shows that people die of different diseases in different parts of the world. Ideas about causes and cures have changed, but not perhaps in the way in which we might have expected.

D Chart showing percentage causes of death in developed and less developed countries.

Disease or condition	Highly developed countries (%)	Underdeveloped countries (%)
Diseases of early infancy	6	22
Other infectious diseases	4	21
Senility (old age)	3	16
Respiratory diseases (connected with lungs)	6	15
Communicable diseases	2	12
Heart disease	39	5
Cancer	18	3
Accidents	6	3
Brain diseases	14	2
Tuberculosis	2	1

Questions

1 a Use pictures **A** and **B** to explain how technology has affected medicine in this century.
   b What is the difference between X-rays (picture **A**) and ultrasound (picture **B**)?
2 Read document **C**. The article suggests we can do things to stay healthy. What do you think those things are?
3 How far has medical science come in the 20th century? Looking at the evidence on these two pages, make two lists:
   a areas of medicine in which great progress has been made this century, and
   b areas of medicine in which great progress has not been made this century.
4 Look at chart **D**, then read the unit on Public health – a world view (page 72) How does that unit help us understand why so many people die of infectious diseases in the underdeveloped world, yet so few die of those diseases in the developed world?

AIDS - new disease, old problems

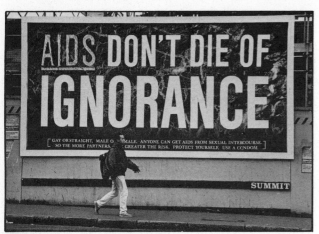

A Government poster, 1987.

All the articles are from 'New Internationalist' magazine, March 1987. This magazine is interested in world affairs and how they affect rich and poor countries.

As you read the evidence, think about how people's ideas about diseases have changed and how much progress has been made.

B By Charles Gregg.

"
'Unclean, unclean', the leper mumbled and rang his bell. Society demanded this warning, on pain of death. And both peasant and lord shrank back, from an illness they didn't understand and couldn't cure. The search for scapegoats, during the Middle Ages, was malicious. The ideal scapegoat should be: (a) different, (b) unpopular, and (c) defenceless. Lepers fitted the bill nicely during the Black Death, but they were few in number. Jews, however, were everywhere in the French province of Languedoc, and were blamed for the Black Death. Lepers were accused of poisoning the wells after being bribed by the Jews who, in turn, were paid by the king of Grenada. This idea led to the slaughter of Jews throughout Europe.
"

C By Graham Hancock.

"
AIDS still remains truly terrible – a fatal infection which is spreading rapidly and which the best minds of modern medical science have been entirely unable to come to grips with. This is the sense in which much ado is certainly *not* being made about nothing. We have learned to live with other diseases and effectively to control most of them. We have not learned to live with AIDS. By the time we have a vaccine or a cure it will have killed tens of millions, devastated economies and changed the universe that we inhabit.

AIDS hurts the poor more than the rich. In underfunded African hospitals and rural clinics the virus is being spread by the practice of reusing needles and syringes which, in better economic circumstances, would be disposed of after each injection.
"

D By Reba Linder.

"
'God can heal everything, including AIDS,' preaches an Anglican Minister in a Nairobi church. 'If we pray and trust, God will heal.'

In another part of town, Ahmed Mohammed, a Muslim healer, scans the Koran. He believes that the Holy Book contains a cure for every disease; if he studies it hard enough, he'll find the answer to AIDS.
"

E By Mark Powall.

"
If more research – between countries, between research institutions and between individual scientists – fails to develop, then a 'cure' for AIDS will remain as far off as it is now.
"

Questions

1 Read documents **B** and **G**.
   a What similarities are there between the ways in which people reacted to AIDS in the 1980s and the Black Death in the 14th century?
   b Why do you think people reacted in a similar way to these diseases?
2 Read document **C**.
   a How serious does the author think AIDS is, and what might its effects on the world be?
   b Why might African countries suffer worst of all?
3 Look at map **F**. The 'New Internationalist' says that AIDS is not only an African disease. Does the map support this view or not? Give examples from the map to support your answer.
4 Read document **G**. Why might people believe that AIDS is spread by casual contact?

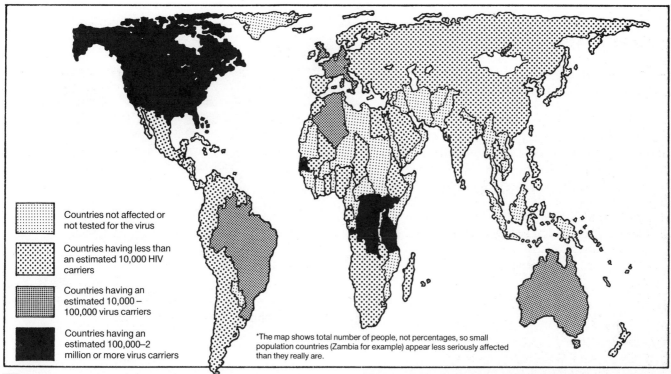

F Estimated carriers of the AIDS virus.

Legend:
- Countries not affected or not tested for the virus
- Countries having less than an estimated 10,000 HIV carriers
- Countries having an estimated 10,000 – 100,000 virus carriers
- Countries having an estimated 100,000–2 million or more virus carriers

*The map shows total number of people, not percentages, so small population countries (Zambia for example) appear less seriously affected than they really are.

One of the articles from 'New Internationalist' talked about the 'myths' that some people believed. Document **G** is one of those myths, something that is not true but that many people believe.

Wordbox

malicious   nasty
devastated   destroyed
underfunded   not enough money
institutions   laboratories in factories or universities
myth   a legend or story
contagion   infection

Myth THREE

AIDS is spread by casual contact – shaking hands with an infected person, sharing cutlery with an infected person, coughs and sneezes, from toilet seats, etc.

The Damage: This myth has had a profound effect on the emotional climate of society, causing a great deal of unnecessary anxiety, suspicion and unhappiness. In America, Australia and elsewhere, there have been cases of children with AIDS (usually contracted through infected blood transfusions) being banned from attending school for fear of infecting others. Where schools have allowed children with AIDS to attend, parents of other pupils have withdrawn their children. Similarly there are fears that AIDS can be contracted from sharing a swimming pool with an infected person. Even the practice of communion in church services has been tainted by the myth of casual contagion – in many churches today communicants will no longer drink from the common chalice.

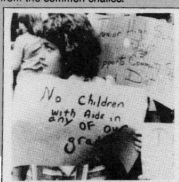

G From 'New Internationalist'.

Questions

5 Document **E** suggests that governments and scientists need to co-operate more to cure AIDS. Read the unit on modern medicine (page 32–33) and suggest reasons why they don't.

6 Document **D** suggests that religion can help in the fight against AIDS. Read the unit on faith in the modern world and suggest reasons why these ideas make sense to so many people (see pages 100–101).

7 The title of this unit is 'New disease, old problems'. Explain what you think this means and what it tells us about the way in which things change in history.

Discovering the body : 1

When you look at the evidence given in the next five units, think about the answers to these questions:
(a) what changes took place,
(b) in which periods did a lot of change take place,
(c) and why did change take place?

Today, doctors have to study for many years before they are fully qualified. They have to pass exams in anatomy (to show they have knowledge about the parts of the body), and physiology (to show they know how the body works). Besides going to lectures and studying books, they have to study skeletons and dissected corpses, so as to find out as much as possible about the complicated workings of our bodies. However, things have not always been like this.

Prehistoric people
In the unit on prehistoric medicine we saw that a cave painting showed what appeared to be the animal's heart (see page 6). Look at picture **A**. It was done in 'X-ray' style. The way the body is drawn may give clues about what the primitive tribes knew about anatomy.

The Egyptians
Archaeologists found beautiful coffins in the tombs of the pharaohs and other important Egyptians. Inside the coffins were the bodies that had been preserved for thousands of years. The internal organs – brain, lungs, spleen etc. had been carefully removed and stored in canopic jars (see picture on page 12). These organs were cut out of the body but could not be cut up and examined in more detail because they would be needed in the next world. The body itself had been soaked in a chemical called liquid natron for 70 days and then wrapped in bandages that had been soaked in resin. The face was covered in a death mask. This had to be as near a perfect copy of the person's face as possible, so the soul could recognize its body in the next world.

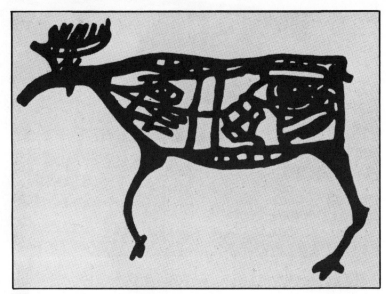

A Tribal X-ray aboriginal painting.

Wordbox

anatomy   the structure of the body
physiology   how the body works
dissected   cut into pieces
natron   a chemical for preserving bodies

Questions

1 How much do you think prehistoric man knew about anatomy? Explain your answer.
2 Match the 'causes of change' in Egypt (column **a**) with the results they brought (column **b**). Copy column **a**, then put column **b** in the correct order.

a Causes of change	b Results
Economy: The Egyptians were farmers.	They had a chance to pick up useful ideas and new information from abroad.
Communications: The Egyptians traded with other countries.	They had to find out more about the organs of the body, so as to preserve the bodies of the dead.
Religion: The Egyptians believed in life after death and mummified important people.	They made bronze tools and instruments – which were an improvement on what had been produced before.
Technology: To build pyramids the Egyptians needed better technology.	Because they didn't have to spend all their time hunting, they could live in one place and educate themselves in skills.

The Greeks

The Greeks questioned previous ideas about the world and produced many new explanations – not just in science but in many other areas. Men like Hippocrates challenged the old superstitious beliefs about disease and put forward that illness might have 'natural' causes and cures, Writers, like Aristotle, studied animals and used their results to work out how the human body worked. At Alexandria, in the distant corner of the Greek empire, men dissected human bodies. However, this was soon banned, because it was thought to be a disgusting and ungodly thing to do. Knowledge then continued to be gained by the dissection of animals. Aristotle thought that it was the heart, not the brain, which was the centre of our thinking. Artists and sculptors showed the body in a lifelike way. The Romans copied and used some of the Greeks' best work. Indeed, the statue pictured below is a Roman copy of an earlier Greek statue.

Claudius Galen

The Romans conquered the Greeks and took their best doctors. One of the best known of these Greeks was Claudius Galen. He studied at Alexandria and went to Rome to seek his fortune. He had gained valuable experience by treating the wounds of injured gladiators, as seen in picture **C**. Galen also treated rich people and healed more than one emperor. He wrote many books about medicine and these became accepted as the truth for over a thousand years. We know that some of Galen's ideas were incorrect; for example, he thought that man's jaw was, like that of many animals, made of two bones, whereas we now know that it is just one bone.

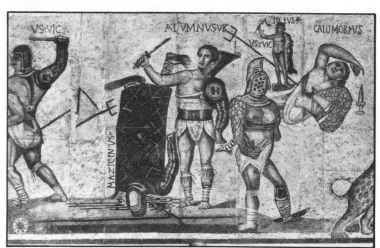

C Treating wounded Roman gladiators.

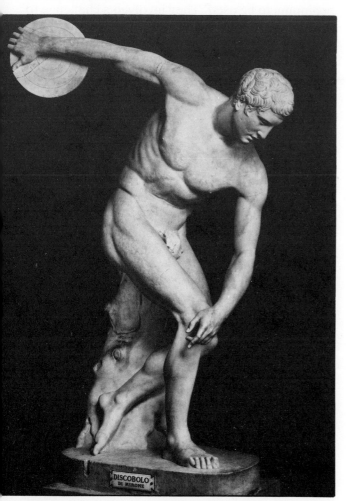

B Statue of a Greek discus-thrower.

Questions

3 Copy these ideas about Greek anatomy and write a sentence to explain whether each of them made the Greeks' understanding of the body better or worse.
   a *Science:* Hippocrates said that illness was not the work of the gods, but had 'natural' causes and cures.
   b *Personal factors:* Some brave men, risked dissecting human bodies.
   c *Religion:* It was said to be against the will of the gods to cut up the body, so human dissection was banned. Galen cut up pigs, rather than humans.
   d *Art:* The Greeks produced superb paintings and statues of the human body.
   e *War:* Greek doctors like Claudius Galen were given the job of treating wounded gladiators.
   f *Education:* Greek doctors, like Galen, wrote many books.

Discovering the body : 2

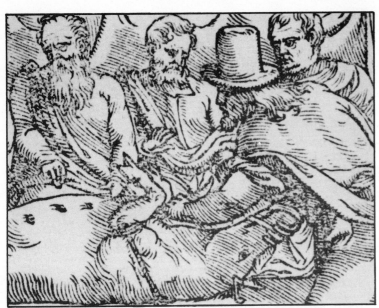

A Galen carrying out a dissection of a pig (from a 16th-century picture).

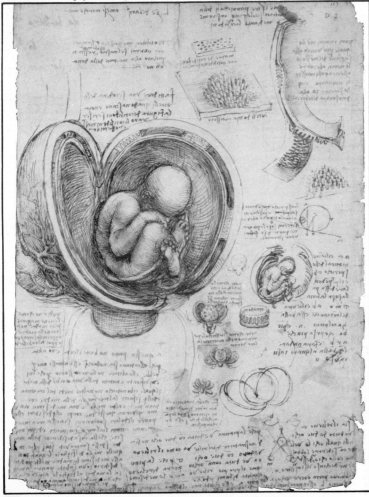

B Leonardo's picture of a foetus in the womb.

Anatomy in medieval times

If some of Galen's ideas were wrong, why were they accepted and not challenged for so long?

Why was there so little change and so little progress for over 1000 years? Well, after the collapse of the Roman empire many of the ideas of the Greeks were 'lost' or ignored. The books of Galen lay hidden in monasteries for centuries. When they were finally translated into Latin – then the language of learning – Galen's ideas began to be accepted by the church. To question Galen was to go against the church.

Galen, as we have seen, had experimented by dissecting animals, not people. The Pope, in 1300 AD, banned the cutting up of corpses. The books of Galen were read aloud in medical lectures, and the study of nature was not encouraged.

Eventually, progress was made in anatomy and physiology. As in other areas of medicine, this progress came about in the Renaissance period. New, more scientific methods of enquiry were beginning to be used. They involved a challenge to the power of the church and a questioning of the ideas of Galen. A new approach towards art can be seen in pictures **A, B,** and **C**. The man responsible for some of the improvements in the knowledge of anatomy made during this period was Andreas Vesalius.

Andreas Vesalius (1514–1564) and new ideas about anatomy

Vesalius was born in Brussels and studied medicine in Paris. He became Professor of Anatomy at Padua University in Italy when he was only 23. He benefited from progress being made in Italy in art and science at the time by people like Leonardo da Vinci. The natural world was being studied and pictures became much more lifelike. By carefully studying the human body, da Vinci improved his pictures. He was even prepared to run the risk of angering the powerful Catholic church, by daring to dissect human bodies. Evidence of this new attitude can be found in the pages of da Vinci's notebook. He wrote 'Do not be sorry that you are giving knowledge through the death of a fellow creature. Do not be prevented by feeling sick, or by sight of those battered corpses, horrible to look at. If you have the art of drawing and the sense of perspective, do not be put off from the task of dissection.'

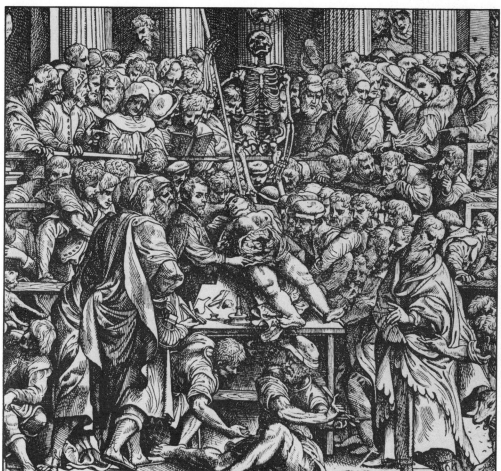

C Vesalius carrying out a dissection, 1543.

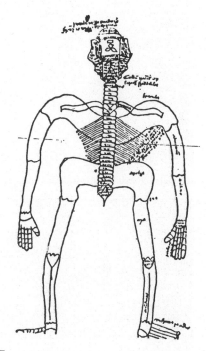

D Medieval picture of a skeleton, 1495.

Vesalius followed da Vinci's example and began to dissect human bodies (picture **C**). So as to get the bodies he had to take a few risks! He stole bodies of executed criminals from the gallows, took the bones apart and soaked them in vinegar. He then took them back to the university and built up a skeleton to study. He even took bones from graves! Once Vesalius began to study the body, rather than read Galen's books, it became clear that a number of Galen's ideas could not possibly be correct. Vesalius showed that the human breastbone was not in fact like that of the ape. He proved that the hip bone was shaped differently from that of the ox. However, Vesalius was strongly criticized, and many people refused to believe that Galen could be wrong.

Despite all this, Vesalius improved our knowledge of the skeleton (see picture **D**). When, in 1543, his book 'The Fabric of the Human Body' was published, students gained the benefit of Vesalius' great drawings.

Questions

1 Why was medieval knowledge about anatomy so poor? Copy these sentences and explain why each was important.
   a *Science:* There were few medical schools.
   b *Communications:* Roads had fallen into disrepair.
   c *Religion:* The church banned dissection.
   d *Technology:* Before the discovery of printing, books had to be copied by hand.
2 If the ideas of Vesalius were good, why were people opposed to them?
3 What problems do people trying to introduce new ideas face? Think of the stories of Leonardo and Vesalius.
4 How did changes in art during the Renaissance help bring changes in medicine?

William Harvey

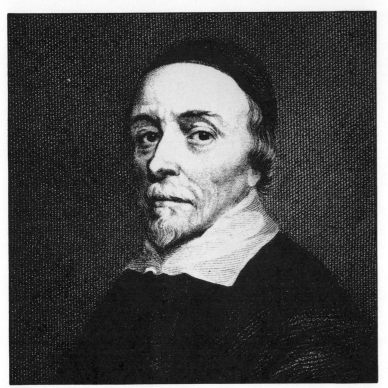

A William Harvey (1578–1657).

If you have been in a laboratory for a science lesson and carried out a scientific experiment, you will have been using similar methods and working in the same way as some of the great scientists of the past. This means that you will have done four things:

a observed the facts,
b built up an idea or 'theory',
c tested the theory by doing an experiment, and
d written down your results or 'conclusions'.

This might seem an obvious thing to do. We call it the 'scientific method'. However, things haven't always been done this way.

In the Middle Ages people learned about the body by listening to lectures from professors. In the lecture the professor would read aloud from the books of the Greek doctor, Claudius Galen. This might have been a good thing to do if all of Galen's ideas had been correct. Unfortunately, the story of Vesalius (page 59) shows that some of Galen's ideas were wrong. Vesalius began to use scientific methods to show that the old ideas were wrong and to prove his own ideas about anatomy. He worked in an anatomy theatre like the one shown in picture **B**.

Questions

1 Draw a simple sketch diagram of the anatomy theatre (picture **B**). Underneath it explain why the anatomy theatre was a better way of finding out about the body than listening to one of the lectures about Galen.

2 Compare pictures **C** and **D** and read about Galen. What mistakes had Galen made about the way the heart works?

3 **a** Copy the four sentences **a**, **b**, **c** and **d** about the scientific method (page 60).
   b Look at the unit on Vesalius (page 59). Write four sentences to show how he used scientific methods to find out more about the body.

4 Look at the unit on Galen (pages 57–58). How do the following things help explain why his ideas about the heart were wrong?
   a the religious laws in those days, and
   b the way Galen did his experiments.

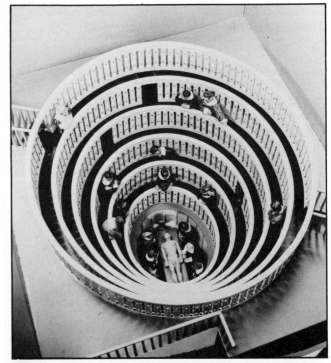

B The anatomy theatre at Padua University, Italy.

People from all over Europe came to Italy to learn about the new scientific method. The unit on the Renaissance (page 28) showed that these scientific methods were being used to find out about many subjects besides medicine. Galileo, for example, was using a telescope to look up at the stars and understand the planets. Vesalius was using science to look down into the body.

One of the people who went to study at the anatomy theatre in Padua was an Englishman called William Harvey (1578–1657). He had studied at Cambridge and had come to Padua to learn about anatomy from a man called Fabricius, who had designed the anatomy theatre. Fabricius had burnt Galen's books and told his students to use scientific methods. William Harvey used those methods to improve our understanding of physiology. Most importantly, Harvey was among the first to discover that the blood circulates around the body.

Picture **C** shows that there are two sides to the heart. Galen knew that there was blood in each side of the heart, but he wrongly thought that the blood flowed from the right side to the left through little holes in the wall called the septum.

When you remember the religious laws in Galen's time, and think about the way he did his experiments, you may understand why he got it wrong. He also made the mistake of thinking that the blood was somehow burnt up in the tissues of the body and remade in the liver.

Picture **D** is a simplified diagram of the heart, taken from a modern biology text book. It shows that the heart is a sort of machine that pumps blood round the body.

Wordbox

septum   a wall between the two sides of the heart
anatomy theatre   a place where students watched a professor cut up a body

D Diagram showing how the heart pumps the blood.

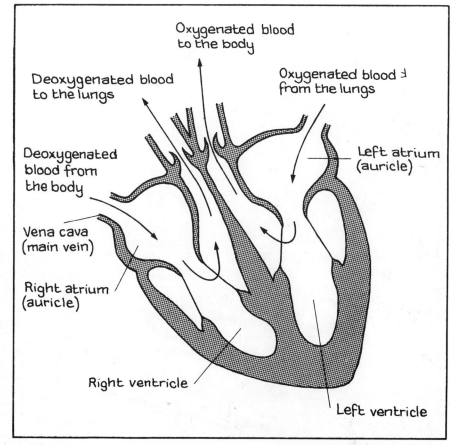

C Diagram showing Galen's wrong idea about the heart.

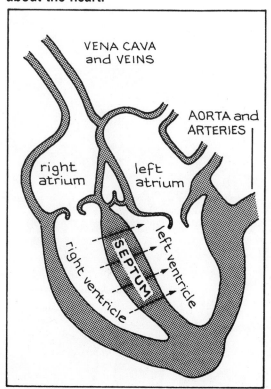

A scientific revolution

Just because some of Galen's ideas were wrong, it doesn't mean he wasn't a clever man, or that he wasn't important. Indeed we have seen how his ideas affected the way many people thought about medicine for over 1500 years. So why was it William Harvey, and not Galen, who worked out that the heart was like a pump?

Harvey lived during a period in which lots of new machines were being built. He observed and studied them and used his understanding of how they worked to help him understand how the heart worked. For example, Harvey looked at these machines and worked out that, although many of them seemed to work with just one quick action – like a water pump (see picture **A**) – they were, in fact made up of lots of actions, all working together. Dr Jonathan Miller, in his book called 'The Body in Question' (1979), thinks that 'Galen could not see the heart as a pump because these machines did not become an important part of the scene until long after his death.'

In other words, it's hard to see that the heart is like a pump if you don't really know what a pump is or how it works.

Harvey tested his idea that the heart was like a machine by examining the way it worked. At first, when he looked at the heart, he found that it moved so quickly that it was hard to be sure how it worked. So he tested his ideas by looking at cold-blooded animals, like toads, frogs and snakes, which had slow-moving hearts. This helped Harvey see that the heartbeat was in fact a set of actions all working together. He described the heartbeat: 'These movements take place one after the other, but so rhythmically that both seem to happen together and only one movement can be seen.'

This idea seemed to make sense when Harvey read about other machines. A book written in 1615 by Solomon de Caus described how pumps worked. 'The pump is easily understood: there are two valves, one below to open when the handle is lifted up and to shut when it is down and another to open to let out the water.'

All Harvey needed to do was to carry out another experiment on the human body to prove his theory that the blood was pumped round the body. This has been called one of the most famous experiments in all the history of medicine and it can be seen in picture **C**.

If you bandage the arm, its valves can be seen on the veins (shown as G, O and H in picture **C**). If you push the finger away from the heart, from one valve to another (from G to O), the space between the two valves will empty of blood. So

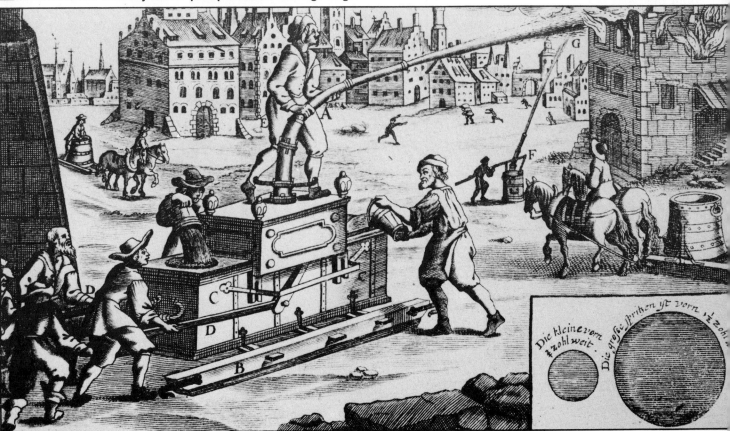

A Seventeenth century water pump used in fire fighting.

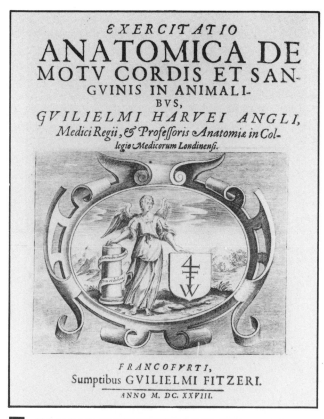

B *(Above)* **The title page from Harvey's book, 'An Anatomical Account of the Motion of the Heart and Blood in Mammals' (1628).**

the blood was going round the body in one direction. It wasn't being mysteriously burnt up.

Harvey's discoveries didn't mean that everyone suddenly stopped using old ideas such as blood letting. However, he had shown that scientific observation and experiment could be used to disprove ideas that people had believed in for thousands of years. These methods were spread across Europe in printed books like the one seen in picture **B**. Science had arrived in medicine!

Questions

1 Explain how each of these factors helped to improve understanding of the way the heart works:
   a technology (pumps), and
   b communications (printing).
2 Look at the information in this unit again. Then read the four sentences about the scientific method (page 60). Write four sentences to show how Harvey used scientific methods to find out more about the heart.

C *(Below)* **Diagrams from William Harvey's book showing how the blood travels through the veins of the arm.**

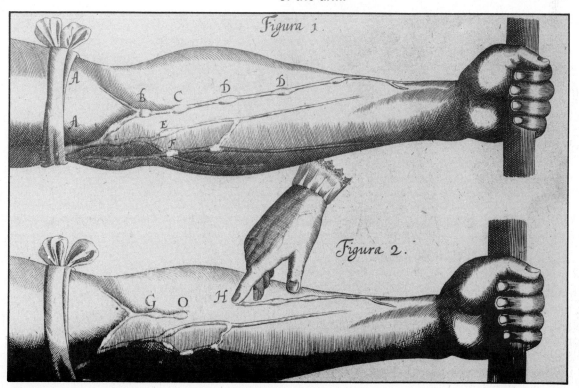

Wilhelm Roentgen and X-rays

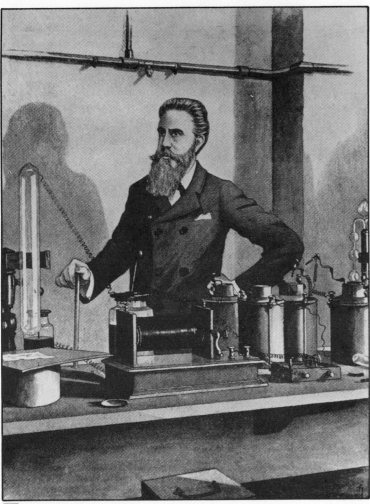

A Artist's impression of Professor Roentgen working in his laboratory at the time of his discovery of X-rays.

A number of machines have been developed during the last century which have greatly added to our knowledge of the body. One of these is the X-ray machine. You may have had an X-ray in hospital or at the dentist's, and will have an idea of why it is such a useful machine.

The person who discovered X-rays was a Dutchman called Wilhelm Roentgen. He became a professor of physics at Würzburg in Germany. Picture **A** is an artist's impression of Roentgen working in his laboratory at Würzburg. It shows him using scientific methods. However, science was not the only factor that was important in helping Roentgen make his important discovery.

One day in November 1885, Roentgen was working in his laboratory. He was carrying out experiments using a long glass tube like the one shown in picture **A**. When electricity was passed through the tube it produced cathode rays. By chance he had left a piece of paper coated with barium platinocyanide on a bench near the tube. The cathode rays left a mark on the paper. When he took the piece of paper into the next room, Roentgen noticed that the mark was still on the paper.

He decided to investigate the matter in a scientific way, and carried out a set of experiments using the paper and these unknown 'x'-rays. When he held his hand in front of a paper screen he found that the rays produced a shadow of the bones inside his hand. So the X-ray could see through the flesh and into the body.

Picture **B** shows the world's first X-ray photograph, of one of the hands of Roentgen's wife. The photograph took 15 minutes to expose and Roentgen's wife was said to have been horrified when she saw it.

Within a year the first X-ray photograph in a hospital had been taken. It was a dangerous business. The operators of the early X-ray machines were exposed to the radiation from the machine for up to 30 minutes every time they took a photograph. By 1922 it was estimated that about 100 of these radiologists had died from exposure to radiation. However, conditions improved, both for operator and patient. Special protective clothes helped cut down the risks of exposure to radiation. More powerful machines were introduced in wartime, and special mobile X-ray units were used by many surgeons in the First World War (1914–1918). The new machines could see the body's organs as well as its bones, and take pictures like that seen in picture **C**.

Wordbox

cathode ray   an electric current
barium platinocyanide   a chemical
radiologist   someone who works an X-ray machine
radiation   a stream of energy that comes from the centre of an atom

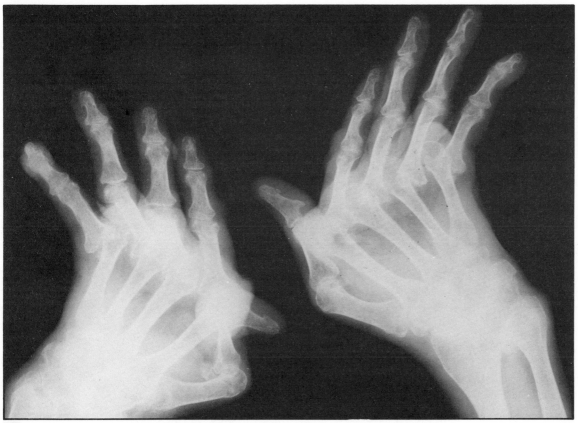

C Modern X-ray photograph.

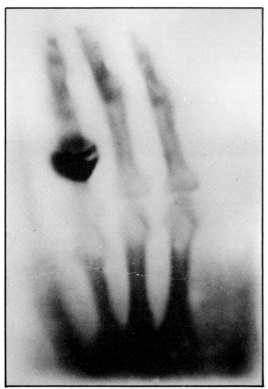

B X-ray photograph of the hand of Roentgen's wife, December 1895.

Questions

1 What do X-rays do and why are they so useful to doctors, dentists and surgeons?
2 How important do you think each of these factors was in the story of X-rays:
   a chance,
   b scientific methods, and
   c war?
3 a Look at picture **A**. Is this a primary source or a secondary source? Explain your answer.
   b Is a secondary source always less helpful to an historian trying to find out about the story of X-rays?
4 Compare pictures **B** and **C**. How much progress has been made in X-ray photography? Describe what you see in these two pictures in your answer.
5 Look at the story of William Harvey (pages 60–63). Harvey was a clever man, but he couldn't discover X-rays. Why not?

Changes in public health : 1

1 Sometimes change does not come about quickly. Things do not always change for the better. Look at the evidence on the next four pages and compare public health in Roman and medieval times. You could fill out the chart on the right. Look at the pictures and writing, then write as much as you can under each heading. Look for similarities and differences. Try to decide whether things had changed for the better or worse.

Aspect of life	Roman public health	Medieval public health
a How the towns were planned		
b Streets		
c Water supply		
d Drains and sewers		
e Toilets		
f Baths		
g Houses		

A Changes in public health through the ages.

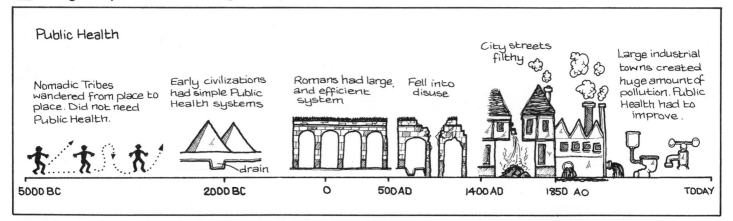

Public Health

Nomadic Tribes wandered from place to place. Did not need Public Health.

Early civilizations had simple Public Health systems

drain

Romans had large and efficient system

Fell into disuse

City streets filthy

Large industrial towns created huge amount of pollution. Public Health had to improve.

5000 BC   2000 BC   0   500 AD   1400 AD   1850 AD   TODAY

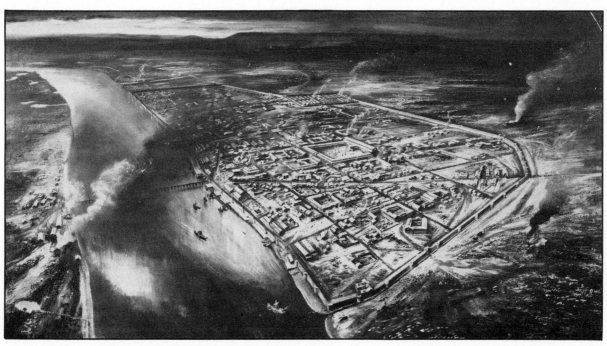

B Reconstruction drawing of Roman London.

66

C From 'The Roman Imperial Army' by G Webster, 1979.

"

In sanitation the Romans used their engineering abilities. Drains and latrines were constantly flushed with the overflow from the water supply, making it a complete system. Trouble was taken to seek out a large supply of water at a spring, and carefully planned aqueducts led it to the town, which was sometimes several miles away. Drains discharged into rivers at points well below all watering points for animals, and when this was not possible there were large soak-aways which worked much like the modern septic tank. Where the site of the town was on a hill and such arrangements were impossible, water tanks were constructed below ground.

"

E Archaeological report by Professor Bosanquet published in 'The Universal History of the World'.

"

In drainage and plumbing the modern world has not greatly surpassed Roman methods. Lead water pipes were found under the floor of the house of Livia on the Palatine Hill, Rome. Almost every private house had its main service pipe with cisterns and taps.

The Cloaca Maxima, Rome's oldest and longest sewer, is a great paved and vaulted tunnel which exists into the River Tiber. It is still used today and is so big that boats could pass through it.

"

F From 'The History of Drainage and Water Supply' by Dr Fielding Garmson, 1929.

"

Until the fourteenth century the water supply of Hamburg was mainly by hand buckets. Then a system of supply through hollow logs from wells was begun. These well systems only supplied part of the town and only the lower floors could be supplied. The water leaked away and was poor in quality.

"

Wordbox

sanitation cleaning for health
aqueduct a bridge carrying water
septic tank sewage treatment tank
vaulted arched

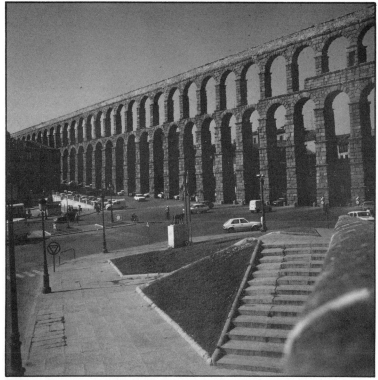

D The Segoria Aqueduct, built by the Romans in Spain.

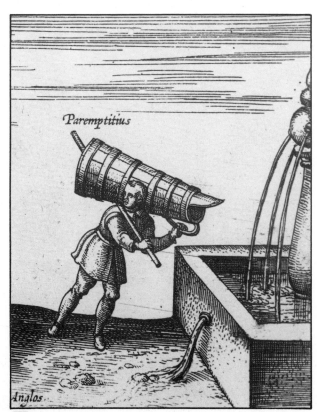

Paremptitius

G An apprentice fetching water, 1572.

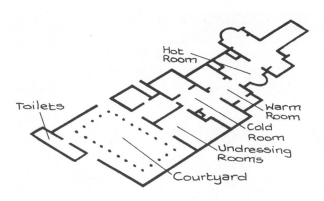

B Plan of the Roman public bath house at Silchester (redrawn).

A From 'English Social History' by G M Trevelyan, 1942 (describing early morning in Edinburgh in Medieval times).

"

Far overhead the windows opened, five, six or ten storeys in the air, and people of Edinburgh emptied the collected filth of the last twenty-four hours into the street. It was good manners for those above to cry 'Gardy-loo!' (Gardez l'eau) before throwing. The person down below cried back 'Haud yer han', and ran with humped shoulders, lucky if his vast and expensive full-bottomed wig was not put out of action by a torrent of filth.

"

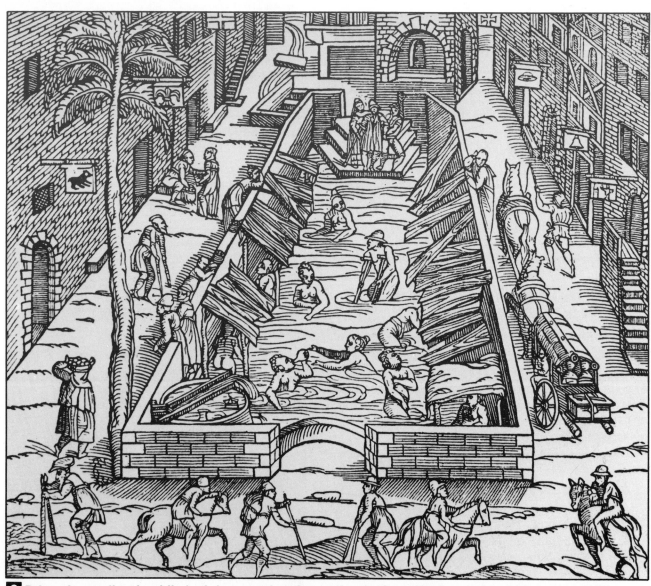

C Print of a medieval public bath house taken from a book about Venice, Italy, published in 1553.

In Roman Timgad there were 15 public baths, as well as many well built public toilets. One of the toilets had 26 carved stone seats, each enclosed by stone dolphins. Its drains were kept constantly flushed by a fountain in the centre.

D **A letter from the Roman writer Seneca.**

❝

We think ourselves poor if our walls are not covered with huge mirrors, if our ceilings are not buried in glass and our swimming pools lined with marble, and if the water does not pour from silver spouts! And I am talking only about the baths of the common people.

❞

It is interesting to note that it was once said of Queen Elizabeth I: 'She doth bathe herself once a month, whether she require it or not.' This may not be surprising when we read document **E**.

E **Description by Sir William MacArthur of the body of the murdered Archbishop of Canterbury, Thomas à Becket, 1170.**

❝

The dead Archbishop was clothed in an extraordinary set of garments. On the outside was a large brown mantle, next a white surplice, underneath this, a fur coat of lambs' wool; then a woollen pelisse; below this the black robe of the Benedictine order; then a shirt; and finally next to the body; a tight-fitting suit of coarse hair-cloth covered on the outside with linen. The innumerable vermin, fleas, bugs, lice etc which had infested the dead Archbishop were so active that his clothes boiled over with them like water in a simmering cauldron.

❞

Ideas about personal cleanliness seemed to change slowly, as document **F** shows.

F **Fifteenth-century French book of etiquette (rules of behaviour).**

❝

When you wash your mouth do not spit back into the basin.
Do not spit on the table; it is unbecoming.
Child, if your nose is snotty, do not wipe it with the same hand you use to hold your meat.

❞

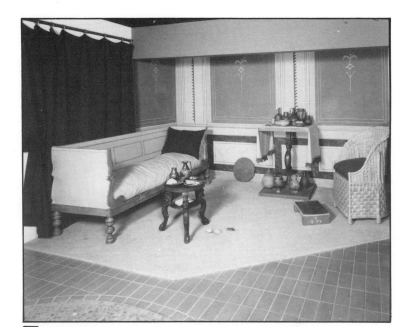

G Model of the inside of a Roman house, based on archaeological discoveries at Silchester.

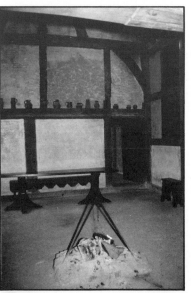

H Photograph of the inside of a wealthy medieval farmer's house, reconstructed at the Weald and Down Open-air Housing Museum, Sussex.

Wordbox

pelisse   a long cloak or coat
Benedictine order   a group of monks
innumerable   a great number
etiquette   manners

Industrialization

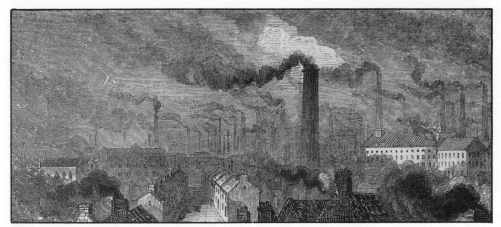

A Picture of Manchester in the middle of the 19th century.

	1801	1851
Bradford	13	104
Glasgow	77	329
Liverpool	82	376
Birmingham	71	233
Manchester	70	303
Leeds	53	172
London	957	2362
Bath	33	54
Norwich	36	68
York	17	34

B Population of towns, 1801–1851 (in thousands).

The cities that sprang up all over Europe as a result of 19th century industrialization suffered as much from plagues as had the cities of the Middle Ages. It was not the Black Death that people feared but cholera, a deadly disease that had its origins in Asia. Its germs were carried in water but it was not until the end of the century that scientists worked this out. By that time it had already killed millions.

Looking at picture **A** you can get some idea why disease spread so quickly in densely populated areas. Table **B** shows how the population in this country had risen in just 50 years. The impact of such a disease on a small industrial town is shown in document **C**. The figures for Bilston are no surprise when you consider the conditions in which many industrial workers had to live.

D From an enquiry into the state and condition of the town of Leeds by Robert Baker, published in 1842.

"

Courts and cul-de-sacs exist everywhere . . . In one cul-de-sac in Leeds there are 34 houses, and in ordinary times there dwell in these houses 340 persons or ten to every house. The name of this place is Boot and Shoe Yard, from whence the Commissioners removed, in the days of Cholera, 75 cartloads of manure which had been untouched for years.

For the most part these houses are built back-to-back. . . A house of this description will contain a cellar, a house and chamber . . .

To build the largest number of cottages on the smallest possible space seems to have been the original view of the speculators. Thus neighbourhoods have arisen in which there is neither water nor privies.

"

CHOLERA STATEMENT.

Population of Bilston, in 1832........ 14.492
No. of Persons attacked by Cholera 3,568
No. of Persons who died by Cholera 745
No. of Widowers who lost their Wives
    by Cholera. 103
No. of Widows who lost their Husbands
    by Cholera 131
No. of Orphans under 12 years of age.....450
The first Case August 3rd.—The last Case
    September 18th, 1832.
Amount of Subscriptions received £8,586

C From a memorial in Bilston, near Birmingham.

Wordbox

industrialization the growth of factories and machines
widowers men whose wives have died
orphans children whose parents have died
subscription money paid
cul-de-sac dead-end street
Commissioners officials
speculators people who invest for financial gain

Cities other than Leeds were no better. Document **E** is about Manchester.

E Extract from 'The Moral and Physical Conditions of the Working Class', 1832, by Dr Kay.

" ——————————————————

The greatest portion of those districts lived in by the labouring population (mill workers) are newly built. . . The houses are ill drained, often ill ventilated, unprovided with toilets, and in consequence, the streets which are narrow, unpaved and worn into deep ruts, become the common resting place of mud, refuse and disgusting rubbish. . . In Parliament Street there is only one toilet for 380 inhabitants, which is placed in a narrow passage from where its flow of muck infests the close-by houses, and must prove a most fertile source of disease.

————————————————— "

What made things even worse was the fact that water was obtained from street pumps which sometimes served hundreds of families. It was here that cholera flourished.

Governments all over Europe were concerned about these outbreaks of disease but weren't sure how to deal with them. Because there were conflicting ideas about how the disease was spread it was difficult to know how to stop it. However, it was clear to many that the terrible housing conditions of the poor must be one reason why they always suffered the most from any outbreak of cholera.

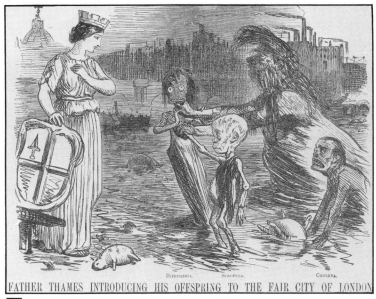

FATHER THAMES INTRODUCING HIS OFFSPRING TO THE FAIR CITY OF LONDON

F A cartoon drawn by John Leech for 'Punch', early 1850s.

Wordbox

ill-ventilated no air
in consequence as a result
fertile plentiful

Questions

1 a What were living conditions like for poorer people in big industrial towns in mid-19th century England? Support your answer with evidence from picture **A**, table **B** and documents **D** and **E**.

  b Explain the connection between these living conditions and the spread of cholera.

2 Look at document **C**.
  Copy and complete these sentences. Explain whether each is true or false.
  a Cholera killed half the population of Bilston.
  b If you got cholera you died.
  c The cholera epidemic of 1832 lasted for 6 months.
  d The deaths from cholera brought about other problems.

3 Look at cartoon **F**.
  Describe in detail what is happening in the cartoon and explain the point you think the cartoonist is trying to make.

4 Read these two pages again, then compare the industrial city with the medieval town. Had there been much improvement in public health? Explain your answer.

5 Look at table **B**.
  a How do you think they gathered the information needed for this?
  b What difficulties might they have had in gathering the information?

A world view

A **Chart showing Acts of Parliament which affected public health in Britain 1906–1946.**

1906 **Education (Provision of Meals) Act:** allowed authorities to help in providing school meals.

1907 **Notification of Births Act:** Medical Officer of Health to be informed of a birth – he could then arrange for a health visitor to call.

Education (Administration Provisions) Act: provided for regular medical inspection and treatment for school children.

1908 **Old Age Pensions Act:** a state pension provided for 70-year-olds.

1909 **Town Planning Act:** set rules for planning and building of houses.

1911 **National Health Insurance Act:** an insurance scheme for the poorly paid so that they could draw benefit when sick.

1918 **Midwives Act:** allowed for payments to trainee midwives.

1919 **Housing Act:** obliged local authorities to provide homes for those returning from the First World War.

1930 **Housing Act:** required moves towards slum clearance.

1946 National Health Service was set up.

New Towns Act: provided for building of new towns away from existing, congested cities.

D **From the annual report of the Director-General of the World Health Organization, 1964.**

"

Seventeen years after the creation of the World Health Organization the control of communicable diseases is still the most important health challenge facing mankind. . . plague is increasing in certain areas; cholera has taken the lives of thousands of people in recent years; smallpox continues to be a major hazard to all nations. . . . Malaria is far from being eradicated. Tuberculosis remains as one of the most widespread infections. There has been a definite upsurge in the incidence of syphilis and gonorrhoea. Yaws still constitutes a major public health hazard in many parts of the tropical and sub-tropical belts. . . The most formidable obstacle to bringing communicable diseases under control, however, is that most of the countries concerned do not yet have adequately functioning public health services.

"

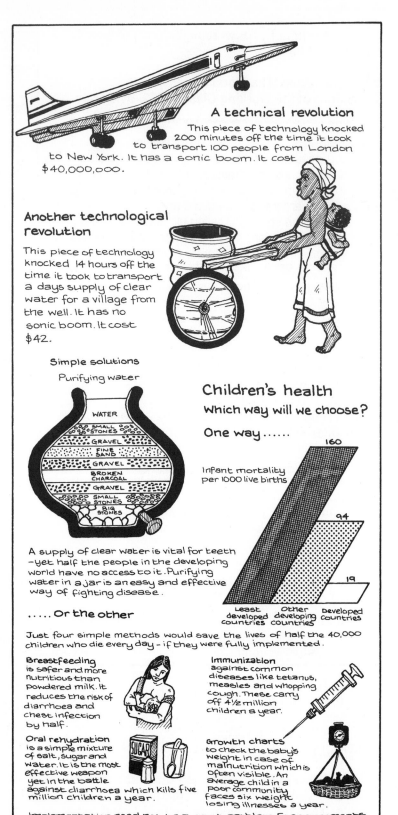

A technical revolution

This piece of technology knocked 200 minutes off the time it took to transport 100 people from London to New York. It has a sonic boom. It cost $40,000,000.

Another technological revolution

This piece of technology knocked 14 hours off the time it took to transport a days supply of clear water for a village from the well. It has no sonic boom. It cost $42.

Simple solutions

Purifying water

WATER
SMALL STONES
GRAVEL
FINE SAND
GRAVEL
BROKEN CHARCOAL
GRAVEL
SMALL STONES
BIG STONES

A supply of clear water is vital for teeth – yet half the people in the developing world have no access to it. Purifying water in a jar is an easy and effective way of fighting disease.

Children's health

Which way will we choose?

One way......

160

Infant mortality per 1000 live births

94

19

Least developed countries | Other developing countries | Developed countries

.....Or the other

Just four simple methods would save the lives of half the 40,000 children who die every day – if they were fully implemented.

Breastfeeding is safer and more nutritious than powdered milk. It reduces the risk of diarrhoea and chest infection by half.

Immunization against common diseases like tetanus, measles and whopping cough. These carry off 4½ million children a year.

Oral rehydration is a simple mixture of salt, sugar and water. It is the most effective weapon yet in the battle against diarrhoea which kills five million children a year.

Growth charts to check the baby's weight in case of malnutrition which is often visible. An average child in a poor community faces six weight losing illnesses a year.

Implementation need not be a great problem. For governments that cannot address the root cause of infant mortality and child malnutrition – that is poverty and inequality – these four simple techniques at least offer an acceptable, apolitical start.

B **Drawings from the 'New Internationalist Calendar', 1986.**

Wordbox

immunization   vaccination
malnutrition   not enough nourishing food
implementation   carrying it out
apolitical   not political

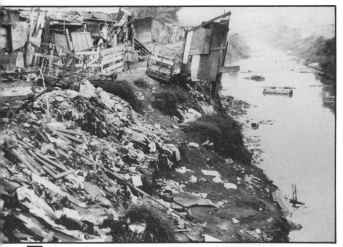

C Slum conditions in Sao Paulo, Brazil.
E *(Below)* **World population growth rates.**

Questions

1 Choose three of the Acts shown in Chart **A** and explain how they helped improve public health in Britain.
2 a Look at document **B**. Concorde is described as a 'technological revolution'. Explain what you think this means.
   b What do you think the author of document **B** is trying to say about technology and public health?
3 Look at map **E**. How does it help us understand some of the other public health problems described on these two pages?
4 a What evidence can you find on these two pages to suggest that much still needs to be done to improve public health worldwide?
   b What evidence can you find on these two pages to suggest that public health worldwide could be improved quickly and cheaply?
5 Compare the evidence in these two pages with that in the unit on page 92. How do the policies of world governments shown in documents **A, B** and **C** of pages 92–93 help explain why public health problems are so great in many 'underdeveloped' countries?

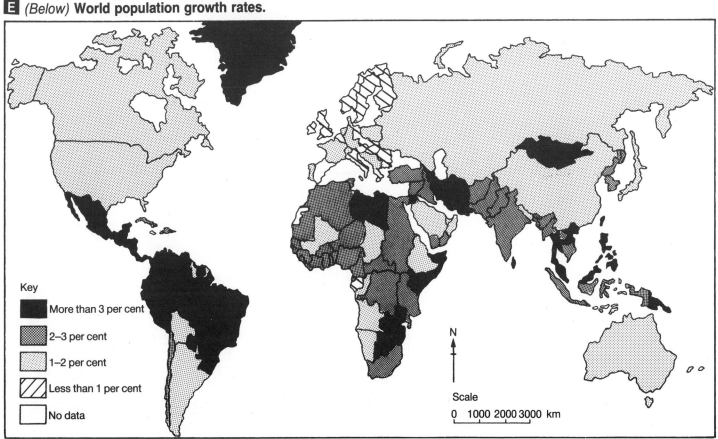

Key
More than 3 per cent
2–3 per cent
1–2 per cent
Less than 1 per cent
No data

N

Scale
0   1000 2000 3000 km

Women in the ancient world

If you were asked to make a list of important women you have learned about in history, and then another list of important men, which list would be longer? Try looking at the index of almost any school text book. How many women have been thought important enough to be included? Why should this be so?

In recent years some writers have begun to fill in the gaps in our knowledge. A historian called Sheila Rowbotham has described how women have been 'hidden from history'. Another historian, called Deirdre Beddoe has given in her book 'Discovering Women's History' some reasons why women have been left out from history. These examples are to do with the ways girls learn about history: 'The teaching of history in schools and universities still presents students with an almost exclusively masculine view of history. . . In school, class exercises reinforce the sex roles; girls are expected to be interested in costume and boys in the navy. Boys are told to write on a day in the life of a Viking/explorer/crusader, and girls about his wife.'

When we look at the history of women in medicine we find that women seem to have been 'hidden' from us.

A Extract from the 'Illustrated History of Medicine' by Albert Lyons, 1979.

"

Women had been healers for a long long time; there were probably female healers in Babylonia, Egypt, Greece, Rome and America. In the Middle Ages the chief medical activities of women were as midwives, but there were also skilful female doctors working secretly or openly. Many of the women in medicine were wives or daughters of surgeons. Although we may see a part played by women in medicine throughout history we may also note that they were disapproved of – and not only by the male physicians. The advance of women into medicine was slow.

"

Wordbox

midwives women who help when children are born
mosaic a picture made from small coloured tiles
woodcut a way of making a picture
exclusively masculine only about men
reinforce the sex roles emphasize male or female aspects

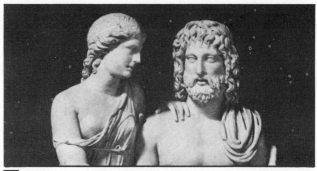

B Statue of Asklepios and Hygeia.

So we don't know much about many of these women healers, and the evidence isn't always easy to understand. Picture **B** shows the Greek healing god Asklepios and his daughter Hygeia. Asklepios had two sons and six daughters. All of the children were healers and the different types of medicine came from the children. For example we get our word 'hygiene' (cleanliness) from his daughter Hygeia. When we looked at the story of Asklepios (page 16), we saw that the god's temple was a sort of hospital, where many patients were treated. But how important a part did women play?

C From 'The Story of Nursing' by D Edwards-Rees (1965).

"

Yet for all the fame of the six daughters of Asklepios it is not certain that there were women nurses at the temple. There were priestesses at the altars, there were women who directed the work of the bath attendants, there were midwives.

But on the whole, it is thought that women were of no great account among the Greeks.

"

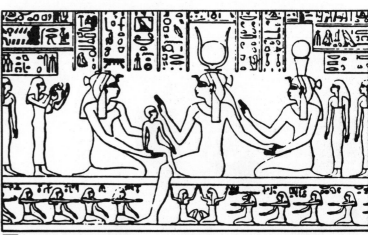

D Wall painting from the temple of Dendera, Egypt.

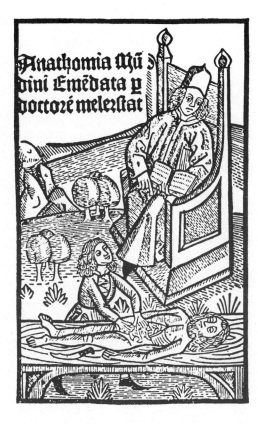

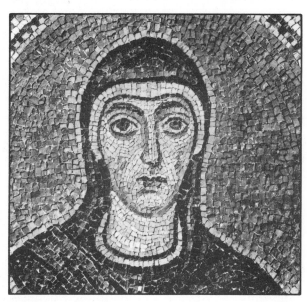

E *(Left)* **The woodcut front cover of a book about anatomy, 1493.**

F *(Below)* **Mosaic of about 500 AD. It shows St Felicity of Carthage, patron saint of sick children.**

Questions

1 **a** Look at the questions in the first paragraph and answer them.

   b Do you agree with what Deidre Beddoe says about girls and history? Think about your own history lessons for examples.

2 Look at evidence **A**, **D**, **E** and **F**. In what areas of medicine do women seem to have been involved?

3 Copy out the following statement and explain whether you think it is true or false. Give reasons for your answer: 'The person shown cutting up the body in picture **E** is a woman.'

4 On pages 74 and 75 we have used different sorts of evidence. The four pictures are very different, but each can be useful to the historian. Copy and complete the chart to work out how useful they are.

5 Having looked at the pictures on these two pages, do you think the way in which a picture is made affects its usefulness to the historian? Mention things seen in the pictures in your answer.

	Statue (Picture **B**)	Wall painting (Picture **D**)	Woodcut (Picture **E**)	Mosaic (Picture **F**)
a What has this piece of evidence got to do with women?				
b Why was this piece of evidence written or made?				
c What does this piece of evidence tell us about women in medicine?				

Women in the Middle Ages

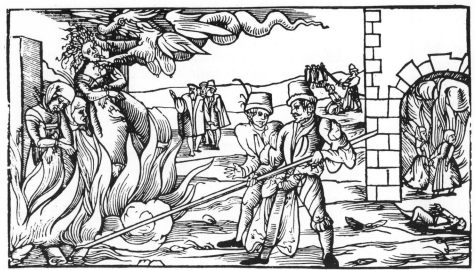

A *(Left)* **A witch being burned, from a German book, 1555.**

Why was it that women didn't hold important positions in medicine in the Middle Ages? Why don't we hear of women surgeons and physicians from that time? To answer the questions we need to know more about women's rights and women's position in the world in the Middle Ages. We must remember that the Christian church was very powerful in western Europe in the Middle Ages. People listened to what the priests had to say about how people were to behave. Men controlled the church. Women were not allowed to be priests.

The historian Patricia Morison has written that many of the poorer people in the Middle Ages would not have gone to physicians or surgeons for medical help, but to the local 'wise woman'. She would have known a lot about herbs and common-sense treatments for medical problems. Unfortunately, we still don't know much about these women because most of them couldn't write. Also, history books were written by men. Nevertheless, although many men couldn't write we still know about their history. A few books, called 'herbals', have been found. These contain the sorts of herbal recipes that the wise women would have used. The church was suspicious of these women, and decided that many of them were witches. The Belgian physician, Johann Wier, wrote a book in 1563 about women who were 'ignorant, wicked and boast of medical knowledge that they do not have. They tell lies to the common people who come to them for advice about all sorts of medical problems. They are not ashamed to say that the illness was caused by witchcraft and spells. It is these women who come from the devil.'

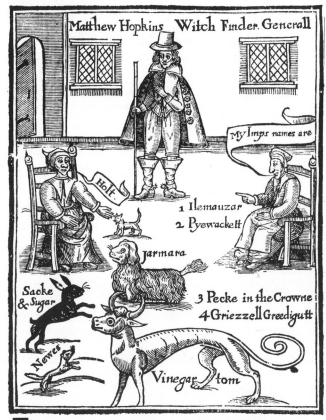

B The front cover of a medieval book called 'The discovery of witches' by Matthew Hopkins.

Wordbox

engraving a way of carving pictures
herbalist a person who knows about the power of herbs
ointment a soft mixture used in medicine

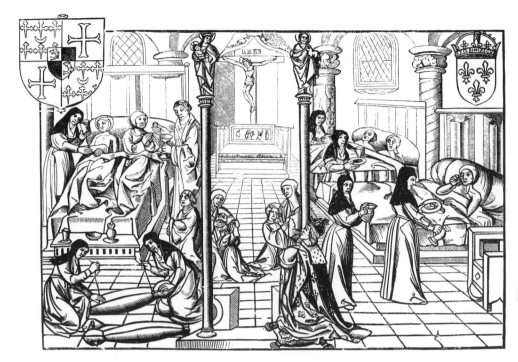

C A 16th century wood engraving, showing the 'hotel dieu' in Paris.

Arab women were involved in medicine. We know that there was an Arab medical school at Salerno in Italy. Women doctors were amongst those who studied there. This was very different from the way in which women were involved in medicine in Christian Europe. We may understand one of the reasons for this difference when we read something from the Islamic holy book, the Hadith. 'When the Holy Prophet (peace be on him) went forth to battle he was accompanied by his wife, Ummi Saleem and a company of women from among the Ansar who provided water and tended the wounded.'

One of the most famous of the Arab women doctors was called Trotula. She was famous throughout Europe, as we hear in this description by a French herbalist. 'I belong to a lady who is called Madame Trot of Salerno: Know that she is the wisest lady in all the four quarters of the world. My lady sends us into different lands . . . to kill wild beasts in order to extract good ointments from them, to give medicine to those who are ill in body. . .'

However, although women became doctors there isn't much evidence to suggest that they were allowed to be surgeons.

In Christian Europe some women joined the church and became nuns. Monasteries and nunneries were important in the treatment of the sick in the Middle Ages. Picture **C** shows nuns at a hospital in Paris called the 'hotel dieu'.

Questions

1 From picture **A**, what do you think happened to witches?
2 a Why do you think it was easy to accuse wise women of being witches?
  b Why do you think the church might want to accuse wise women of being witches? Pictures **A** and **B** might help you.
3 a What did Johann Wier, the Belgian physician, think about women in medicine?
  b Do you think that the people who drew pictures **A** and **B** would agree with Johann Wier's ideas about women? Back up your answer by mentioning things from the pictures.
4 Is there any evidence to suggest that Arab women were treated differently from Christian European women? Explain your answer.
5 Compare the conditions in the medieval hospital, picture **C**, with that seen in Florence Nightingale's hospital (page 79). What changes seem to have taken place?

Florence Nightingale

When we read about war we see that although battles kill and wound people, they also bring changes in medicine. Sometimes these changes are for the better, sometimes for the worse. Wars have made a difference to the position of women in medicine. In this unit we shall see how the work of Florence Nightingale was connected with what happened in the Crimean War, and how some important changes in nursing came about.

Before we look at the work of Florence Nightingale it is useful to remember that, until the 19th century, much of the nursing was done in the home. Many of the nurses were badly paid, untrained, poorly educated and even drunken. The Middlesex Hospital Committee realized that something needed to be done. A meeting in 1838 decided 'We hope that by raising the wages we will get and keep the better kind of nurses – women who will take more interest in the way they work, behave and dress.'

Cartoon **A** shows what some people thought about nurses at that time. However, not much was done until 1853, when Britain and France went to war with Russia.

William Russell wrote a horrifying report which shocked the readers of *The Times* in England. The report said that the sick were dying at an average of 80 a day. Hospital ships were packed with as many as 500 badly injured men, with only two surgeons to look after them and almost no water to drink. In one hospital at Scutari there were over 1000 patients suffering from diarrhoea and only 20 chamber pots to go round. There was an inch of

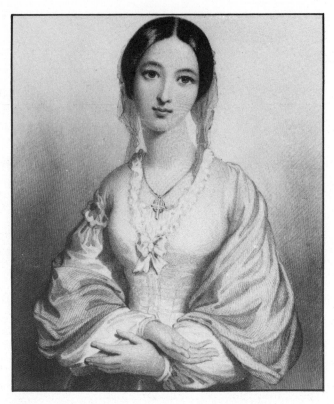

B An engraving of Florence Nightingale.

liquid filth covering the floor, and the soldiers had no shoes or socks. Their food was left in the muck. Half of all the men suffering from diarrhoea did not survive. There were no screens, so the surgeons amputated the legs of soldiers in front of the rest of them.

A rich, well educated English girl called Florence Nightingale was so disgusted by what she read that she decided to do something about it. She got help and money from the Secretary for War, Mr Sidney Herbert. She arrived in the Crimea on 5 November 1854 with 38 nurses. However, at first, the army doctors refused to help her. But conditions were so desperate that the army couldn't stop Nightingale's nurses from getting down to work. Picture **C** shows the improvements that were made to the wards. In less than 2 years she had cut down the death rate in the hospital from 42% to 2% of all wounded patients. She returned to England as a national heroine and raised enough money to open a school of nursing. Soon, more schools were set up and large numbers of nurses were trained. In 1830 there had been no trained nurses in Britain; 50 years later there were almost 7000.

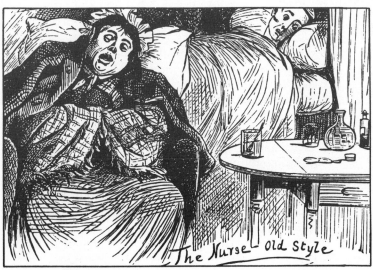

A A cartoon showing a nurse at the bedside of a patient, 1879.

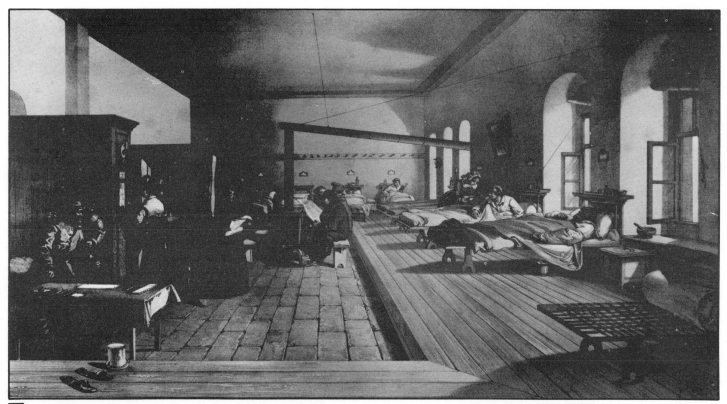

C A hospital ward in the Crimea, showing improvements made by Florence Nightingale, 1855.

Although Florence Nightingale had helped bring changes in medicine, she couldn't change a lot of old ideas – as we see in document **D**.

D Article by a male doctor in the medical journal 'The Lancet' in 1870.

" They are sexually, constitutionally and mentally unfitted for the hard and unending work, and for the heavy responsibilities of general medical and surgical practice. Women might become midwives but in an inferior position of responsibility as a rule. I know of no great discovery changing the boundaries of scientific knowledge that owes its existence to a woman of our or of any race. What right, then have women to claim mental equality to men? "

Wordbox

constitutionally   strong in body
Crimea   part of Russia by the Black Sea

Questions

1 Look at cartoon **A**. What point do you think the person who drew the cartoon was trying to make about the standard of nursing in the middle of the 19th century? (Before the changes brought about by Florence Nightingale.)
2 When Florence Nightingale arrived in the Crimea there was a lot of opposition to her.
   a Why might this seem strange today?
   b What clues are there in picture **B** to explain why the doctors did not want women like Florence Nightingale to work in the conditions of the early hospitals in the Crimea?
   c Using document **D**, suggest other reasons why there was so much opposition to the work of Florence Nightingale.
3 Wars help and hinder medical progress. How much do you think the Crimean War affected the position of women in medicine? Give examples from this chapter to support your answer.
4 Compare the picture of Florence Nightingale's hospital in the Crimea (picture **C**) with William Russell's description of the hospital at Scutari. What changes had been made?

Equal rights ?

How much progress have women made this century in the battle for equal treatment in the medical profession?

A Extract from the 'Illustrated History of Medicine' by the medical historian, Albert Lyons, 1979.

"

So many women have entered the medical profession and made outstanding contributions that you hardly notice which worker is female and which male . . . Women now enter medical schools, become doctors, professors and receive grants for research on an equal footing with men. In Finland, at least half the dentists are women and in the Soviet Union a high percentage of the doctors are women.

But it would be less than accurate to say that females are fully accepted in all fields of medicine. The fields of surgery and orthopaedics have not attracted many women. In most countries there are few women medical directors – except in schools for women.

"

As we saw on the previous page, war can have an important effect on medicine. In both world wars more nurses were needed to cope with the huge numbers of injured soldiers. Poster **B** was issued during the First World War and gives us some important clues about women's rights in those days. Many women who had never previously worked answered the call to help the war effort.

But was this recruitment good for the future of nursing?

C Extract from 'Suffragettes International' by Trevor Lloyd, 1971.

"

Women who had never previously worked did not often go into factory jobs. But many more nurses were needed than before, and many of the new recruits were women from the comfortable classes who felt that they were now doing something useful; it was an unfortunate side effect that their willingness to work for low wages encouraged everybody to think that nursing was a vocation for which a living wage was quite unnecessary.

"

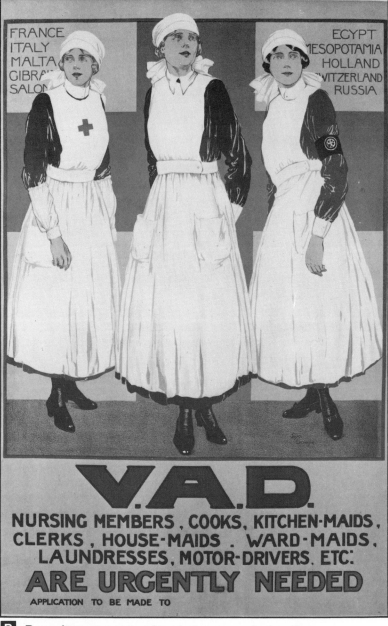

B Recruitment poster aimed at women during the First World War.

Wordbox

orthopaedic	healing children
suffragettes for women	members of a movement for votes
recruitment usually military	getting people to join an organization,

E Nurses taking part in a demonstration in the 1970s.

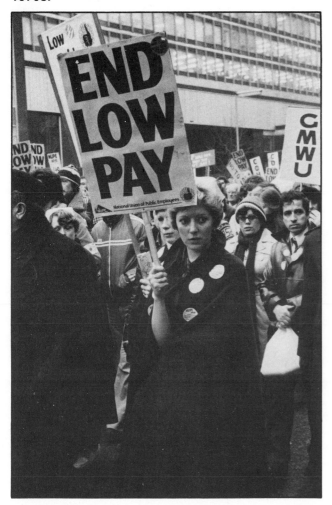

Do girls have equal educational chances at school? They go to 'mixed' schools and can take the same subjects and exams as boys. However, fewer girls go on to colleges and universities.

D Extract from 'In Her Own Right' by Jacky Gillot.

"

Women teachers suffer from the old assumption that girls are good at arts subjects and appalling at maths and science. Consequently there is an increasing lack of good science teachers in girls' schools (with the exception of biology). The result is a lack of good science students. Meanwhile the myth sticks that girls are bad at science – indeed it sticks so hard, that some county education authorities make smaller buildings. . . for laboratories in girls' schools because girls take less sciences!

"

Even though laws have been passed to give equal rights with men, we still find complaints of discrimination. This can be seen in this article by an Asian woman, Dr K Tandon. She describes (document **F**) the problems she found as she tried to become a doctor in England.

F Article from the October 1983 issue of 'Spare Rib', a magazine about women's rights.

"

After completion of one year I was told by my bosses that although I was very competent, general surgery was really a man's speciality and that I would never progress beyond a certain level. They said that the number of fully qualified women general-surgeons in the United Kingdom can be counted on the fingers of one hand – why not be a midwife and deal with women or try eye surgery which is a little like doing embroidery?

"

Questions

1 Look at poster **B**. List the jobs which women were being asked to do. What do most of these jobs have in common?
2 Compare poster **B** and document **C**.
   a What sort of women became nurses during the First World War?
   b What clues are there in the evidence to help explain why nursing became a poorly-paid job?
3 Use the evidence in documents **A, C, D, E** and **F** to write paragraphs explaining:
   a ways in which the position of women in medicine has improved since the First World War, and
   b ways in which the position of women in medicine has not improved much since the First World War.
   Support each paragraph with quotations from the documents.
4 'Women's position in medicine reflects women's position in society.' Explain what you think this means and give as many examples as you can from all the units on women and any other information you may have.

From temples to tower blocks

1 Study the following documents and pictures (and look elsewhere in the book) and look for ways in which hospitals changed through the ages. Then fill in the chart with examples.		What does the hospital look like?	How comfortable would the patients be?	How important did these people think hospitals were?
	Egypt			
	Greece			
	Rome			
	Middle Ages			
	The Industrial period			
	Modern hospitals			

A 'Healing Gods of Ancient Civilisations' (Egypt), by Dr Jayne.

"

There were many healing temples in the valley. Large numbers of people travelled and made annual pilgrimages to be cured by their favourite gods. These healing temples were places of medical knowledge. On the walls were inscriptions to remember cures. Priests and laymen who were to take up healing practised and studied here.

"

D Description of a hospital run by priests in Paris (the hotel dieu) in the 16th century.

"

In one bed lay six sick people, the feet of one next to the head of another, children next to old people, men next to women. In the same bed lay people who had infectious diseases next to people only slightly unwell. Women groaned in childbirth next to typhus patients crazed with fever. The most miserable food was given out in tiny quantities and not at regular intervals. The doors were always open. Anyone could bring anything in. While the sick on one day might be starved, on another day they might get drunk and kill themselves by overloading their stomachs. The whole building swarmed with rats, and the air was so vile in the sick wards that the attendants did not dare enter without a sponge soaked in vinegar held to their faces. The bodies of the dead often lay on the bed for more than a day and during this time the sick had to share that same bed. It was very rare that anyone recovered from a surgical operation. There was only one surgeon for 549 patients. The hospital had only five surgical instruments, which included a trephine for opening the skull and a mouth plug for keeping the jaws separated.

"

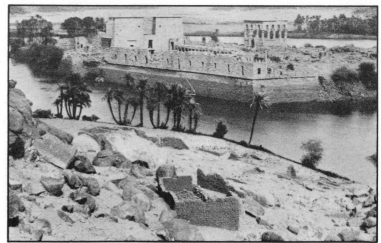

B Temple dedicated to Imhotep, the Egyptian healing god.

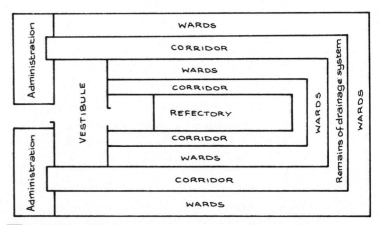

C Plan of a Roman hospital near Düsseldorf in Germany, about 100 AD.

E Picture of conditions in a military hospital in the Crimea, Russia, 1853, before the arrival of Florence Nightingale.

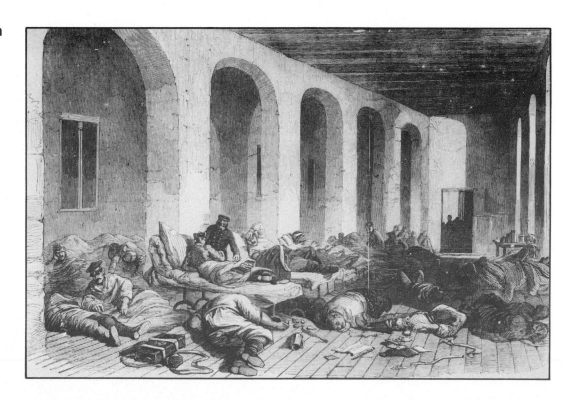

F A new ward, opened in 1984 at the Elizabeth Garrett Anderson Hospital.

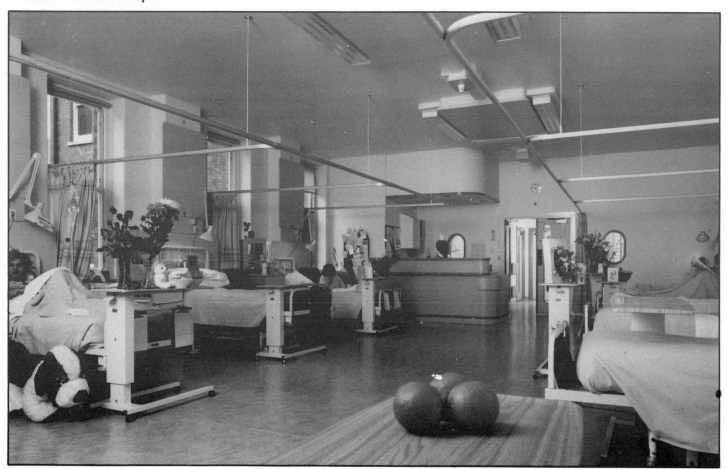

Governments and health

The following units look at important factors that have affected the history of medicine. We have seen how things change, now we need to look at why things change. We are looking for things called factors of change. The first factor we shall be looking at is the part governments play in the story of medicine.

As you look at the evidence in these units, try to think about these points:

(a) when did governments play an important part in medical history,

(b) how easy was it for governments to change people's ideas about medicine,

(c) and why were some people opposed to governments taking charge of medicine?

Governments have not always existed. In prehistoric times, and in groups such as the aborigines, there isn't the need for it. Today, governments of most countries play a big part in the lives of their people. Most important, governments are responsible for the organizing and running of the economy and deciding on what things money should be spent. For example, we have seen that the governments of ancient Egypt, headed by the pharoahs, spent lots of money building huge monuments such as the pyramids.

Not only do they spend money, governments must also try to raise it. This is done by taxing the working population. The tax payers then expect the government to pass laws and generally run the country to protect them and their property. Without the support of the people, governments have always found it hard to rule. Therefore they try all kinds of methods to try to win the support of people

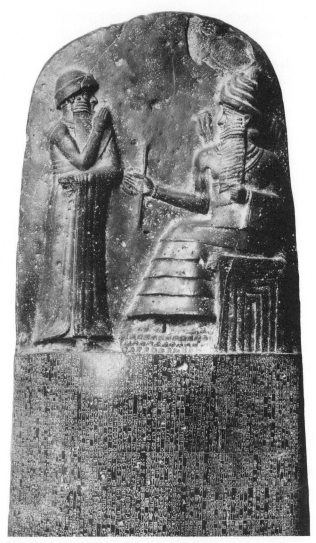

A Monument showing the laws of Hammarabi, about 1800 BC.

B From the Laws of Hammarabi, 1800 BC

"

If a doctor has treated a gentleman with a bronze lancet for a severe wound and has caused him to die or if he has opened with a bronze lancet an abcess of the eye of a gentleman and has caused the loss of the eye, the doctor's hands shall be cut off. . .

If the doctor has treated the slave of a freeman for a severe wound with a bronze lancet and has caused his death, he shall render slave for slave. . .

If a doctor cures the broken bone of a gentleman, or cures a sickness of his bowels, the patient shall give the doctor five shekels of silver. . .

If he is a slave, his owner shall give the doctor two shekels of silver. . .

"

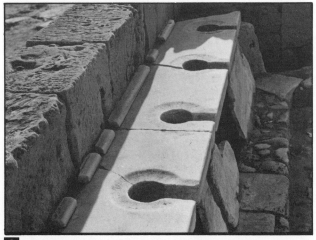

C A view of the interior of a Roman public lavatory, Leptis Magnia, Libya.

Very much later than Hammarabi we find the Roman government spending money on people's health.

D From Julius Frontinus, appointed Water Commissioner for Rome, in 97 AD, by the Emperor.

"

My job concerns not merely the convenience, but also the health, of the city and so this task has always been handled by the most important men in the State.

When M Valerius Maximus and P Decius Mus were consuls, the Appian aqueduct was built. Forty years later the two censors, Marius Curius and Lucius Papirius contracted to build the Old Anio aqueduct with money from the war booty. Two water commissioners were appointed to take charge of this. In order to bring the water into the city on a gentle slope the conduit had to be made 43 000 paces long.

The aqueducts reach the city at different levels so that some deliver water to the high ground and some to the lower ground. Compare such important engineering works carrying so much water with the idle pyramids and the useless, though famous, buildings of the Greeks.

"

E Ministry of Health poster, issued during the Second World War.

Strabo, a Greek geographer, wrote in the first century BC: 'Water is brought into the city through aqueducts in such quantities that it is like a river flowing through the city. Almost every house has cisterns and water pipes and fountains.'

Governments have tackled different problems through the ages, but it has always been important to try to win support. It is no different in the 20th century.

During the Second World War (1939–1945) the British government wanted to encourage parents to immunize their children against diphtheria. A national advertising campaign was started and posters such at that shown in **E** were issued. Deaths from diptheria declined dramatically once the campaign had been started.

Questions

1 Governments affect everyone's life today. Make a list of 8 ways in which the government affects your life.

2 Look at document **B**.
   a How do the laws of Hammarabi affect medicine?
   b Why do you think these laws were made?
   c What problems do historians face in trying to find out about the medical ideas of civilizations like those shown in picture **A**?

3 Use picture **C** and document **D** to explain how and why the Roman government became involved in the health of its people.

4 Governments often have to persuade people to do things.
   a What was the aim of poster **E**?
   b Mentioning things in poster **E**, explain how it gets its message across.
   c What other methods, besides posters, do governments today use to persuade people to do things?

Governments, plagues and people

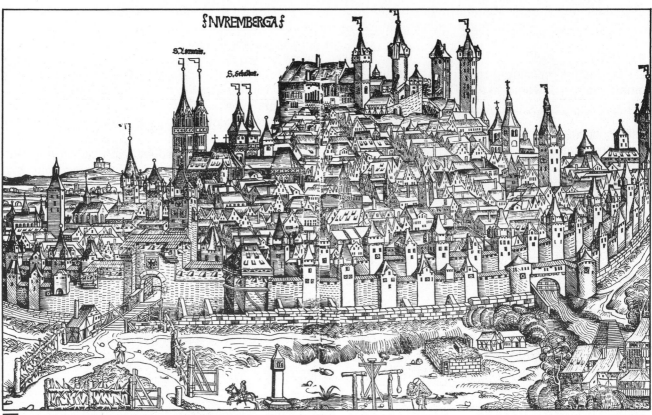

A Nuremberg in 1493, from the Nuremberg Chronicles.

Of all the tasks that confronted governments, some of the most difficult were dealing with outbreaks of bubonic plague or other such diseases. When looking at the evidence in this unit, try to work out:
(a) **how did governments try to fight plagues,**
(b) **did the way governments fought plagues change a lot during the Middle Ages,**
(c) **was the action of governments the only reason why plagues ended, or were there other factors?**

In his book 'Plagues and People' the historian, William McNeill, makes the point that the city governments of Italy between 1350 and 1550: 'responded rather quickly to the challenges presented by devastating disease. Magistrates learned how to cope at the practical level, organizing burials, safeguarding food deliveries, setting up quarantines, hiring doctors and establishing other regulations for public and private behaviour in time of plague.'

Quarantine was a measure introduced by a Venetian official during the 14th century. Because Venice was both an island and an important port, keeping the plague away was vital for its continued success. All visitors were kept away from the city for forty days. If, after this time, they had not developed the plague they were allowed in.

McNeill goes on to make the point that Italian city states were able to do what they wanted because they did not have to ask permission from any superior government or king. In this respect the cities of Italy were lucky. If measures could not be taken quickly and effectively then the population could suffer badly.

To stop the plague spreading and to keep order, some places took drastic steps (document **B**).

In 1665, when the plague struck London, the Lord Mayor decided to take steps to reduce its effects (document **C**).

C **The Lord Mayor of London's rules for the 1665 outbreak of plague.**

66 ▬▬▬▬▬▬▬▬▬▬▬▬▬▬▬▬

Examiners' Office
These Examiner. . . if they find any person sick of the infection, to give order. . . that the house be shut up.

Searchers
Women-Searchers. . . report whether the persons to die of the infection, or of what other diseases.

B A broadsheet showing scenes from the plague in 1665.

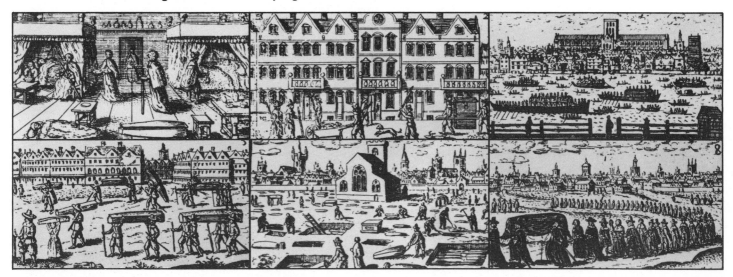

Sequestration of the Sick
As soon as any man shall be found. . . to be sick of the plague. . . he shall. . . be sequestered in the same house, and the house should be shut up for a month.

None to be removed out of infected houses.

Burial of the Dead
The burial of the dead be always either before sun-rising or after sun-setting . . . And that all the graves shall be at least six feet deep.

Every visited House to be Marked
Every house visited, be marked with a red cross of a foot long . . . and with these words. . . 'Lord have mercy upon us.'

"

The measures also told people to clean the street in front of their houses, not to keep pets, and that any dogs in the city were to be killed.

Wordbox

bubonic plague dangerous disease spread by rats
responded answered
safeguarding looking after
quarantine keeping separate and away from certain places
sequestration taking away by order of law

Questions

1 Look at picture **A**, and answer these questions:
  a Why might plague spread quickly in a city like that in picture **A**?
  b What things could the government of such a city do to stop plague spreading through it?
  c In a city like that in picture **A**, who would suffer more from the plague, the rich or the poor? Explain your answer.
2 The Italian cities of the 14th century, and London in the 17th century chose similar methods to control the plague. How do you explain such a similarity?
3 a Read document **C**. How effective would these rules be in stopping the spread of the plague? Try to write a sentence about each of the rules.
  b Are any of the rules mentioned in document **C** also shown in picture **B**? Explain your answer.
4 How valuable is picture **B** as a form of evidence for historians interested in the plague?
5 Use all the documents to explain why governments could do so little to stop the plague in the Middle Ages.

Governments in the 19th century

In industrial areas, disease-ridden conditions remained unchanged because of a number of factors. Doctors could not agree on what caused diseases, and local councils had neither the power nor the money to improve things. Property owners refused to see the need to change and they were supported in this by governments, who thought improvements would be expensive and difficult.

It took fear to change things. The 1831 and 1837 cholera outbreaks so frightened people that investigations began into the health and living conditions of the general public. The most famous study of the nation's health was put together by Sir Edwin Chadwick (1800–1890).

His report, published in 1842, was based on the investigations of doctors, and shocked all who read it (see document **B**).

B Dr Duncan's (Medical Officer for Liverpool) information for Chadwick's Report on the 'Sanitary Conditions of the Labouring Population', published in 1842.

"
. . . finding that not less than 63 cases of fever had occurred in one year in Union Court (containing twelve houses) I visited the court in order to ascertain, if possible, their origin, and I found the whole court inundated with fluid filth which had oozed through the walls from two adjoining ash-pits or cess-pools and which had no means of escape in consequence of the court being below the level of the street, and having no drain. The court was owned by two different landlords, one of whom offered to construct a drain provided the other would join him in the expense; but this offer having been refused, the court had remained for two or three years in the state in which I saw it.
"

Disturbing though the report was, governments, which could have put into practice Chadwick's suggestions, didn't. It took another outbreak of cholera, in 1848, finally to persuade them to act (see chart **F**). Opposition continued. This extract from 'The Times' tries to make a serious point, but in an amusing way.

C Extract from 'The Times', August 1st 1854.

"
The Board of Health has fallen. Mr Chadwick and Dr Southwood Smith have been deposed and we prefer to take our chance of cholera than be bullied into health.

Everywhere the Board's inspectors were arbitrary, insulting and expensive. They entered houses and factories insisting on changes revolting to the habits or pride of the masters and occupants. There is nothing a man so much hates as being cleaned against his will, or having his floors swept, his walls whitewashed, his pet dungheaps cleaned away, or his thatch forced to give place to slate, all at the command of a sort of sanitary bombailiff. It is a positive fact that many have died of a good washing, as much from the irritation of the nerves as from the exposure of the skin no longer protected by dirt.
"

Even in 1892 there were arguments about the cause of cholera, even though Koch had discovered the germ that we now know caused it.

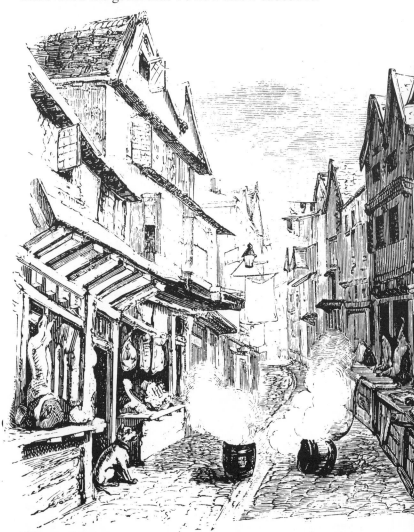

A Tar barrels burnt by order of Exeter City Council to purify the air during the cholera epidemic of 1832.

D Extract from William McNeill's book 'Plagues and People', showing how opponents of public health were eventually silenced.

66

Hamburg in Germany drew its water from the Elbe without special treatment. Next to it lay the town of Altona, where the government installed a water-filtration plant. In 1892, when cholera broke out in Hamburg, it ran down one side of the street and spared the other completely. Since air and earth were identical across the boundary between the two cities, a more clear-cut demonstration of the importance of the water supply in defining where the disease struck could not have been devised. Doubters were silenced; and cholera has, in fact, never returned to European cities since, thanks to systematic purification of urban water supplies.

99

F Chart showing events in public health in Britain, 1831–1883.

1831 Cholera spreading across Europe. Disease reaches Britain and Boards of Health and local Sanitary Boards set up.

1832 Boards closed down because worst of disease is over.

1842 Chadwick publishes his report called 'Sanitary Conditions of the Labouring Population of Great Britain'. The conditions he described shocked many people.

1847 Some local authorities appoint Medical Officers of Health.

1848 Cholera again sweeping across Europe. The British government so worried it passes the first Public Health Act. A Central Board of Health is set up in London under Chadwick. Public health boards could be organized in areas where 10% of ratepayers asked for them, or where the death rate was more than 23 in every 1000 per year. The boards had the power to raise money to pay for drains and sewage disposal and make improvements they thought safeguarded public health.
Dr Snow draws his cholera map of London.

By 1854 182 towns had set up public health boards. But Chadwick's Central Board of Health is closed down.

1855 Board of Health set up again with John Simon in charge.

1864 Factory Act passed making factory owners provide healthier and safer working conditions.

1866 Sanitary Act. Each town to have an inspector to make sure that there are no health hazards in the area.

1875 Public Health Act. Gives local councils power to pull down slums, dispose of sewage, check market places and a range of other public health measures. Each town to have a Health Inspector and a Sanitary Officer.

1883 Robert Koch discovers the germ which causes cholera.

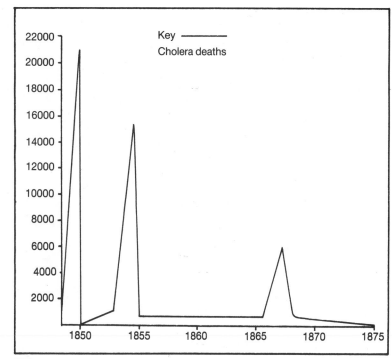

E Diagram showing deaths from cholera, 1845–1875.

Questions

1 Read document **B**. What improvements do you think Chadwick might have suggested in his report? Make a list.

2 Why do you think Chadwick's ideas were opposed? Support your answer with quotations from document **C**.

3 Look at picture **A**. How does it help explain why people were opposed to Chadwick's ideas?

4 Read chart **F**. Which of the things mentioned on the chart was the most important in stopping cholera? Explain your answer.

5 Read chart **F** and look at graph **E**. Did governments pass laws to improve health before or after outbreaks of cholera? Explain your answer by referring to both the chart and the graph.

6 If Koch discovered the cholera germ in 1883, then why do you think people were still arguing about it in 1892? (see document **D**).

7 Using the evidence on these pages, write a paragraph to explain how important you think Chadwick was in the history of public health.

The welfare state

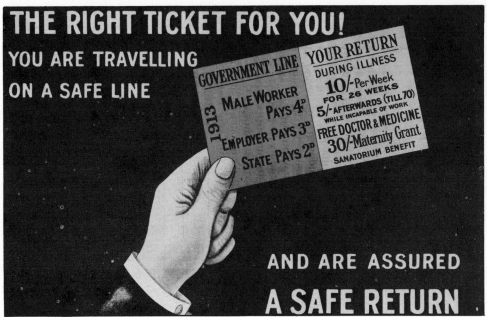

THE RIGHT TICKET FOR YOU!

YOU ARE TRAVELLING

ON A SAFE LINE

GOVERNMENT LINE

1913

MALE WORKER PAYS 4ᴰ

EMPLOYER PAYS 3ᴰ

STATE PAYS 2ᴰ

YOUR RETURN

DURING ILLNESS

10/- Per Week FOR 26 WEEKS

5/- AFTERWARDS (TILL 70) WHILE INCAPABLE OF WORK

FREE DOCTOR & MEDICINE

30/- Maternity Grant

SANATORIUM BENEFIT

AND ARE ASSURED

A SAFE RETURN

A *(Above)* **A Liberal Party leaflet about the National Insurance Act, 1913.**

In the last chapter we saw what a struggle it was for people like Edwin Chadwick to get the government to spend any money or pass any laws on cleaning up towns. Why didn't governments want to get involved in public health? Why did attitudes change? At the beginning of the 20th century there were still no unemployment benefit, sick pay or pensions. You had to pay to go to the doctor.

Slowly, however, governments took notice of the problems of the growing numbers of people living in the towns and cities. More people got the vote, workers organized themselves into unions, and a new type of politician appealed to the mass of the people and promised a better deal for the workers. One of these politicians, called David Lloyd George, put forward an idea to end some of the misery of workers who could not afford to be ill. The idea was called the National Insurance Act. Picture **A** shows how Lloyd George hoped it would work.

National Insurance was an important step forward, but 30 years were to go by before plans were put forward for a national health service which gave equal medical treatment for rich and poor alike. The plans were put forward during the Second World War. The ideas behind these changes can be seen in the following documents.

B From a government film of 1941. A young soldier talks to an older one. (They were played by actors.)

"

We've been doing some hard thinking lately and we haven't got to stop when this job's finished. There'll be work enough, too, when this lot's over, building up something new and better than what's been destroyed. There mustn't be no more chaps hanging around for work what don't come. No more slums, neither. No more dirty, filthy back streets and no more half-starved kids with no room to play in. We've got to pack all them up and get moving out into the brightness of the sun. We've got to all pull together.

"

C Statement by Aneurin Bevan, Minister of Health in the government which introduced the National Health Service.

"

Preventable pain is a blot on any society...

Much sickness and often permanent disability arise from failure to take early action, and this, in its turn, is due to the high costs and the fear of the effects of heavy bills on the family. The records show that it is the mother in the average family who suffers most from the absence of a free health service. In trying to balance her budget she puts her own needs last.

The essence of a satisfactory health service is that the rich and the poor are treated alike, that poverty is not a disability, and wealth is not advantaged.

"

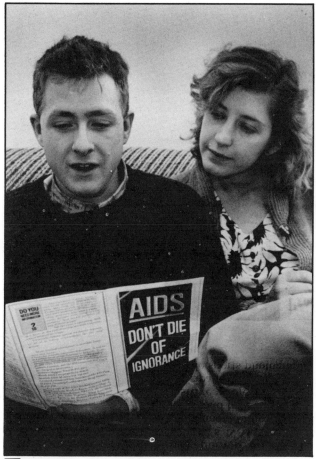

D Young couple reading a Goverment leaflet on AIDS, 1987.

Wordbox

welfare state part of a system of government which looks after the health and well-being of its people

National Health Service free medical treatment for everyone

disability something which holds you back

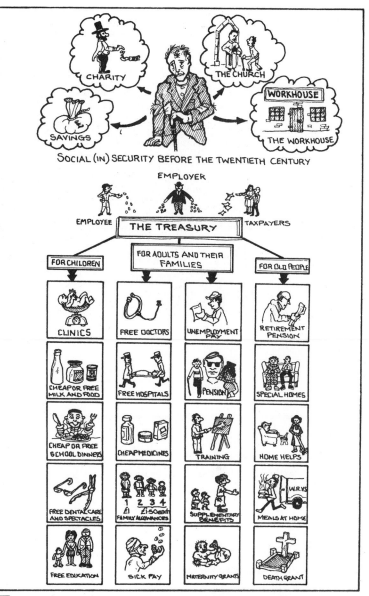

E National health, before and after the start of the Second World War.

Questions

1 Use picture **A** to explain what the National Insurance Act was and how it helped workers.

2 **a** Use chart **E** to write a paragraph to explain what the welfare state does for the people.

   b Why do you think there has been so much change this century?

3 Look at photograph **D**. With a disease like AIDS why is it so important to have a welfare state?

4 The National Health Service seems a really good idea, so why do you think there was a lot of opposition to it when it was introduced?

5 Read these two pages again, then look back at the other units on government. During which century do you think there was the biggest change in governments' involvement in the health of the people? Explain your answer.

A world view

This unit looks at problems of health on a world scale. Read the evidence and think about how successfully governments are dealing with health problems.

RAF lifeline snubbed

Sitting on food for six weeks

THIS picture is a staggering example of how thousands of tons of grain are being stockpiled because of EEC regulations while millions starve.

It was taken at a warehouse near Swindon, Wiltshire, where 100,000 tons of surplus wheat and barley — enough to feed the starving of Ethiopia for six weeks — is heaped high.

Stabilised

The glut this year is so great in Britain alone that the hunt is on for extra warehouses to take in the load.

The Intervention Board has already spent a record £4 million to soak up the excess. This publicly-funded body buys surplus grain from farmers under Common Market regulations to stabilise prices at a time of glut.

'WE DON'T WANT YOUR PLANES'

By ANDREW McEWEN

ETHIOPIA's Marxist leaders yesterday snubbed the British Government's offer of a mercy airlift.

The man responsible for co-ordinating aid for his country's starving millions described plans for the RAF to operate a life-saving shuttle service as 'insignificant'.

Mr Dawit Woulde-Giorgis said: 'We do not want the situation to be exploited by politicians.'

A Article from 'The Daily Mail', 29 October, 1984. Above the article was a photograph of an EEC grain store.

B From 'The Sunday Times', 17 February, 1980.

"

HOW TO AVOID THE THIRD WORLD WAR

The lunacies of Planet Earth.

● The cost of a tank would buy 1000 classrooms; a fighter would pay for 40 000 village pharmacies.

● Half a day's military spending could eradicate malaria, which threatens a billion people.

● The North has a quarter of the world's people, 80% of its income, and 90% of its manufacturing capacity. It consumes 85% of world oil production.

● Since World War II, wars have killed 10 million people in the Third World.

The real world of Willy Brandt:
'Are we to leave our successors a scorched planet of advancing deserts, impoverished landscapes and ailing environments?'

'The abolition of poverty is itself not only a moral obligation. It is against everyone's interests to allow poverty to continue, with the insecurity, suffering and destruction which it brings.'

'Ordinary people in the South would not find it credible that the societies of the North regard themselves as anything other than wealthy.'

"

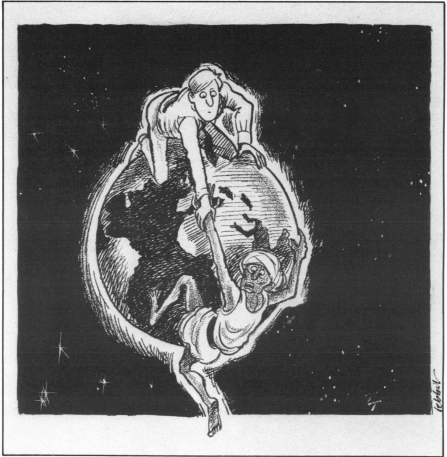

C Cartoon showing how different parts of the world depend on each other.

Wordbox

regulations	laws
EEC	the Common Market
surplus	more than is needed
glut	excess, too much
stabilize	keep steady
Marxist	communist

Questions

1 Look at document **A**. Why might it have shocked many of the people who read it?

2 Read document **B**. What ways are suggested to solve terrible problems like hunger and ill health? Support your answer with quotations from the document.

3 What does cartoon **C** show and what point do you think the person who drew the cartoon was trying to make?

4 a What political point of view does 'The Daily Mail' seem to dislike?

  b If document **A** shows only one point of view, does that mean it is of no value to the historian?

  c What other sources could be used to check 'The Daily Mail's' point of view?

5 Many people agree about how to stop hunger and ill health. Governments want to be popular with the people, so why don't they do more to solve these problems? Suggest reasons.

Religion and medicine

In this unit we will look at how religion affects medicine – in ways which both help and hinder. Perhaps it is hard for some of us today to imagine how important religion was in explaining the world to people who lived in the past. However, when you consider that most of the works of art produced both by primitive tribes and ancient civilizations up to the Middle Ages were to do with religion, this may give you some idea of its importance.

When looking at the evidence about religion, try to think about these points:
(a) at which times did religion have an important effect on medicine,
(b) how much progress did religion bring to medicine,
(c) how much influence did religion have on medicine?

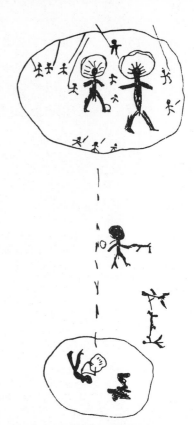

A *(Right)* A Shaman (medicine man) contacting the supreme spirit to help cure a sick member of the tribe. The Shaman is shown at the bottom right, the spirit at the top of the picture.

B *(Below)* A doom painting of heaven and hell, from an English church, 1200 AD.

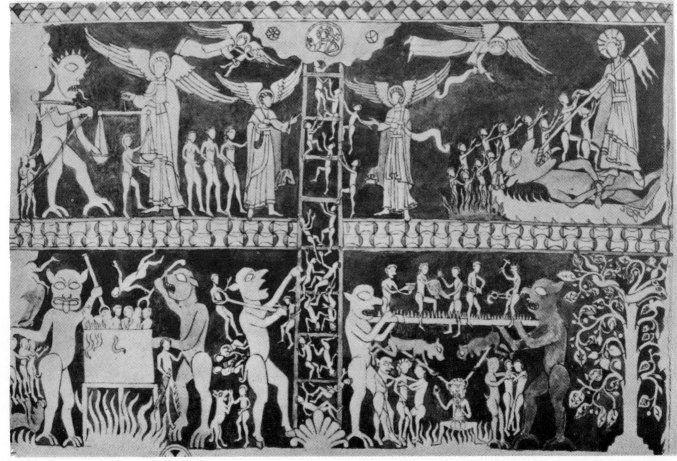

Picture **A** is an example of ancient art; it shows how the gods could be contacted to help the sick.

Picture **B** is known as a 'doom' picture. This is a wall painting from an English church, produced during the Middle Ages. This kind of picture was quite common then.

For centuries, religious ideas provided the only sensible means of explanation to people who did not have a scientific understanding of the world. This was particularly true in the Stone Age. Religion has offered hope to suffering people in the form of faith and prayer. It has also provided another sort of comfort, the healing temples, hospitals, monasteries etc. (see pages 16 and 77).

However, the power of religion has not always been used to help people. For example, many religions would not allow the body to be cut up, and there have been times when people, in trying to help sick people, have been punished by religious groups (see the witch burning, page 76).

Wordbox

hinder hold back
primitive simple, or not very advanced
civilizations people who lived an advanced way of life in cities

Questions

1 Use picture **A** to explain how a medicine man would try to get the gods to heal the sick. Mention some of the problems the medicine man might face.
2 According to picture **B**, what is it like in
   a heaven, and
   b hell?
   Mention as many things as you can from the picture to support your answer.
3 How does picture **B** help explain why the Christian church did not allow the body to be cut up?
4 Why were pictures like the one shown in picture **B** painted on the walls of churches throughout Europe? What were people who saw these pictures expected to think and do?
5 Pictures **A** and **B** come from very different civilizations but they have certain things in common. What?
6 The aim of this chart is to bring together some of the ideas about religion and medicine already mentioned in this book. You are asked to find ways in which religion helps and hinders medicine. Copy and complete the chart, using the page numbers given on the chart. The first one has been done for you. Don't worry if one column is longer than the other or if you can't find examples for both columns.

Religion and medicine through the ages chart

People	Ways in which religion helps	Ways in which religion hinders
Egypt	**a** They were organized into groups of priests, physicians, and encouraged to be clean. **b** They believed in life after death. The pharaoh's body was mummified. They removed the organs from the body. **c** Mummification needed chemicals and drugs. These helped in medicine. **d** They washed their clothes and shaved the body because they thought the gods wanted it. **e** They built healing temples. These were a bit like schools and hospitals.	**a** Gods were thought to cause disease so they didn't look for other explanations. **b** They did not cut up the organs of the body because they were needed for the next world. This made it harder to find out about how the body worked. **c** They tried to solve many medical problems by chanting spells to the gods and by believing in the power of lucky charms.
Greece	(pages 14-17, page 57)	
Rome	(pages 18-21, pages 66-67)	

Islam

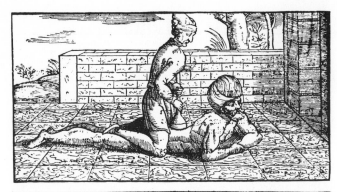

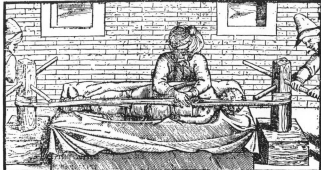

B Pictures from 'The Canon of Medicine', a book by the Arab doctor, Avicenna.

Wordbox

the ancients   the old doctors
empire   a large area controlled by one group of people

About 1200 years ago a group of Arabs began to spread the ideas of the Islamic religion far beyond the holy city of Mecca (see map C). The sayings of the prophet Muhammad in the Islamic holy book, the 'Hadith', offered millions of people a way of explaining the world. These sayings of the prophet give us an idea of the way in which Muslims (followers of the prophet) were expected to behave.

When looking at the evidence in this unit you should try to work out:

(a) in what ways did the Islamic religion help medical development,

(b) in what ways did the Islamic religion hinder medical development,

(c) did any Greek or Roman medical ideas continue in Islamic medicine?

A Parts of the Islamic holy book, the 'Hadith'.

"

The Holy Prophet (peace be on him) said: Cleanliness is half of Faith. Keep your houses and yards tidy. God does not like dirt and untidiness. Brushing the teeth cleanses the mouth and pleases God. He who does not trim his nails and his moustache is not one of us. He who goes to sleep while his hands smell of food has only himself to blame if harm comes to him. Every Muslim must have a bath once a week, when he must wash his head and the whole of his body. Do not put up a sick man and a healthy one together. If you hear of the plague keep away from it. If the plague breaks out in the area where you are, do not leave.

"

C Map showing the spread of Islam.

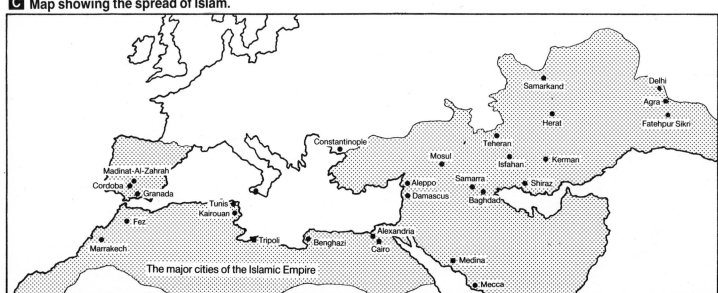

The major cities of the Islamic Empire

The Islamic religion taught that education was very important, as we see in picture **B** and in the book by an Islamic writer (document **D**).

D From 'The Cultural Side of Islam' by Muhammad Pickthall.

"

The Muslims set out on their search for learning in the name of God at a time when Christians were destroying all the learning of the ancients in the name of Christ. The Christians had destroyed the library at Alexandria. Learning for them was only for the devil and unbelievers. The priests publicly burnt the books of the Greeks and Romans.

However, the educated men of Islam set to work on the translation of the ancient books. So the Muslims saved the ancient learning from destruction and passed its treasures down to modern times. The Greek contribution to medicine would have been lost without the efforts of the Muslims.

"

The Muslims built up the medical school at Alexandria and set up new schools throughout the Arab empire. Medical schools, built all over Europe in universities like Oxford and Cambridge, were based on the Arab schools. A paper-making factory was set up in Baghdad. The ideas of the Arabs were written down in books.

The Greek and Roman ideas were included in a medical textbook written by a Persian doctor called Avicenna. His book was written about 1000 years ago and was used by medical students for hundreds of years. It was one of a large number of Arab books which were translated into Latin and read in many European countries. It is thought that his book was read by Vesalius, who made an important contribution to medical progress (see page 59).

Another Arab doctor, called Rhazes, wrote many medical books, in which he described the knowledge needed to become a good doctor. He gave information about diseases such as smallpox and measles.

Islamic doctors did not approve of some of the old medical ideas that were still used in Christian Europe – as we see in this Islamic medical book: 'It is a foolish custom to have blood let out of the body when it is not needed. . . The expert physician has no need to choose times for blood letting. To test this with horoscopes is a vain idea.'

Islamic surgeons were experts at treating eye complaints. Some of them used alcohol as a disinfectant. They didn't know about germs and therefore couldn't understand why wounds became infected, but the surgeons found that the alcohol helped heal the wounds. Their religion would not allow the body to be cut up, so Islamic surgeons couldn't make much progress in anatomy or physiology. Many patients died from the cautery iron, which was a red-hot bar used to seal wounds. Christian surgeons copied this idea (see page 36). Islamic religion ordered that male and female patients should be kept separate. Hospitals were built with separate wards for men and women – as well as separate wards for people with different diseases. Good standards of cleanliness were kept up in these hospitals and well trained doctors looked after their patients.

Questions

1 What did the prophet say about the plague (document **A**), and why was this good advice?

2 Why do you think Arab hospitals were so clean? Quote evidence from document **A** to help you answer the question.

3 Read through these two pages again and find examples to show how the Islamic religion both helped and hindered medicine.

4 Look at the chapters on medieval medicine (page 24) and medieval surgery (page 25). Which ideas do you think were 'borrowed' from Islamic medicine?

5 Compare map **C** with the map of the Roman empire on page 18.
   a Can you name any countries both empires conquered?
   b Do you think having a large empire might help or hinder medical development? Give reasons for your answer.

Christianity in the Middle Ages

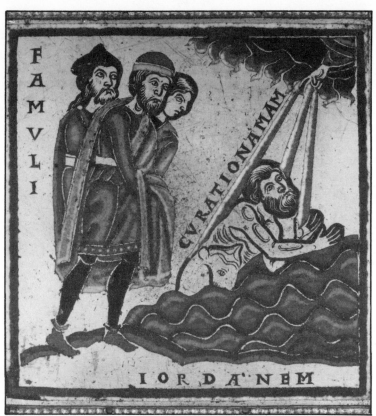

A 'The healing of Naaman', a picture made in **1180.** The words mean that Naaman is healed in the River Jordan.

As you read the evidence in this unit, ask yourself these questions:
(a) how fair is it to say that the Christian church held back progress in medicine,
(b) some Medieval ideas seem strange to us, why did people hold these ideas?

After the great doctors of the Greek period, and the clean towns of the Romans, we arrive at the Middle Ages and everything seems to get worse. Towns and streets seem to be filthy (page 66–67), knowledge about art and the body seems to get worse (pages 58–59).

It is suggested that the Christian church held back progress. But things aren't quite as simple as that.

In his book 'The Body in Question' Dr Jonathan Miller tries to improve our understanding of medicine in this period by suggesting that the Christian church was more interested in the spirit and the next world than in the body and this world. So it seemed less important to study nature, art and science than it did to study what life was about. If the next world could be a paradise, then it did not seem to matter much if you did not live long in this life.

If you look at the pictures drawn in the Middle Ages – for example the skeleton (page 59) – it is easy to think that artists were not very good at drawing at this time. However, you have to think about the reason why these pictures were drawn. Picture **A** was not drawn so as to be accurate, lifelike or realistic, it was drawn for a religious reason.

The Pope was the head of the Christian church. He issued orders about how people should behave. These orders tell us about the ideas of the church in the Middle Ages and help explain what medicine was like in those days (document **B**).

B From a decree by Pope Boniface VIII, 1300.

"

It is forbidden to cut up the bodies of the dead. This abominable savagery, stupidly adopted by some people, should from now onwards be abolished. Now this is not only abominable in the sight of God, but extremely revolting under every human respect. This is inhuman and unholy and must be eradicated. We order that wherever the Catholic faith is followed, this or any other similar abuse of the bodies of the dead should stop for ever.

"

Almost everyone went to church in the Middle Ages. People's ideas about the world were influenced not only by the pictures they saw on walls or stained glass windows, but also by what they were told in the Bible (document **C**).

C Part of the Gospel According to John, chapter 5, verses 2–4.

"

Now, there is at Jerusalem by the sheep market a pool, having five porches. In these lay a great multitude of sick folk, blind, withered, waiting for the movement of the water. For an angel went down at a certain season into the pool and touched the water; whoever then stepped into the water was cured of whatever disease he had.

"

Wordbox

saint a holy person
abolished ended
eradicated destroyed
consult go to see somebody about something

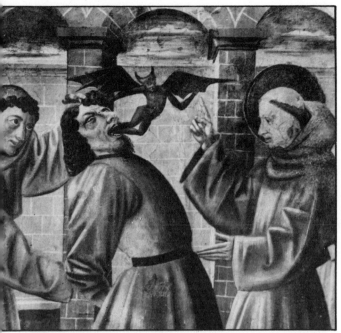

D **A wall painting in the church of St Francis, at Montefalco in Italy.** It shows a man being healed by St Anthony.

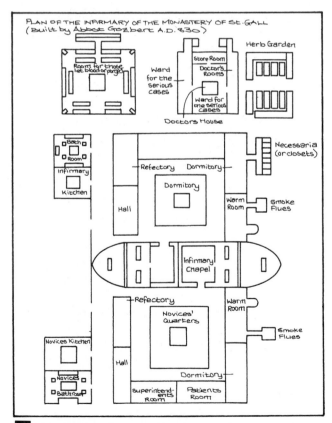

E **Plan of the hospital of the monastery of St Gall, built in 830 AD.**

Since saints were said to be so powerful, their words were taken seriously. Saint Jerome in the 4th century AD believed that, in order to be close to God and obey God, a person should have nothing to do with things of the body. This included washing. He wrote: 'Does your skin roughen without baths? Whoever is once washed in the blood of Christ needs not wash again.'

Some religious people followed his ideas. This may also have affected people's opinions about physicians. A churchman called Gregory of Tours declared that: 'It is against God's will for the sick to consult earthly physicians instead of going to the tomb of St Martin. Because disease comes from God's anger an appeal to the saints works better than the drugs of the physician.' Monks and nuns carried out their religious duties to help the sick. Monasteries were places of medical importance – as can be seen in picture **E**.

Questions

1 a What does picture **A** show and why do you think it was painted?
  b The people painted in picture **A** do not look very lifelike or realistic. Does this mean that the painters of the Middle Ages were not very good? Explain your answer.
2 Read document **B**. Why do you think many people in the Middle Ages thought that it was wrong to cut up the body? Support your answer with quotations from document **B**.
3 Read document **C**. Why do you think it made sense to believe in miracle cures in the Middle Ages?
4 Look at picture **D**. Describe what is happening in the picture and explain what it tells us about people's ideas about the cause and cure of disease in the Middle Ages.
5 a Look at picture **E**. Find as many things as you can to do with medicine in the picture.
  b Do you think the monks of St Gall (picture **E**) would agree with the ideas on medicine put forward by Gregory of Tours? Explain your answer.
6 Read through these two pages again and fill out a 'Christianity in the Middle Ages' column of the 'Religion' chart started on page 95. Find examples to show how Christianity both helped and hindered medicine.

Faith in a modern world

The 20th century has seen fantastic changes in science and technology. However, this does not mean that religion has not played an important part in medical history in this century. Look at these documents and try to decide how medicine has been affected by religion. What do we learn about the way in which ideas about medicine continue or change throughout time?

A Article in 'The Daily Telegraph', 5th January 1978.

"

New respectability for traditional African healing methods was predicted yesterday after a decision by the Kingdom of Swaziland to give 'witch-doctors' the same status as western-trained medical men. The Swazi decision is expected to be followed throughout Black Africa and is linked to a resolution by the World Health Organization to broaden its definition of health care. . . Swaziland's lead has been followed by Zambia where a move is under way to give witch-doctors professional status. Nigeria has also decided to build a joint school of traditional medicine and a normal teaching hospital in Lagos.

"

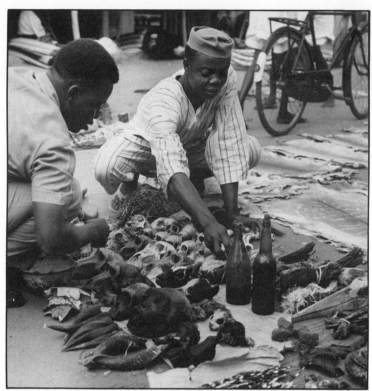

B A 'traditional' doctor selling his goods in Dahomey, West Africa.

Jehovah's Witnesses
Blood transfusions are acceptable to many Christian groups but to some, like the Jehovah's Witnesses, the giving of blood is thought to be wrong. One of their books gives advice to Jehovah's Witnesses about this problem, especially in situations where they are questioned about the use of blood transfusions: 'You might reply: "The newspapers have published stories about some situations in which they felt that Witnesses might die if they did not accept blood. Is that what you have in mind?. . ." Jehovah's Witnesses say they actually benefit from better medical treatment because they do not accept blood. "In the case of a patient that refuses blood, are there any alternative treatments?"

'Often simple saline solution, Ringer's solution and dextran can be used as plasma volume expanders, and these are available in nearly all modern hospitals. Actually, the risks that go with use of blood transfusions are avoided by using these substances.

The issue here really is loyalty to God. It is God's word that tells us to abstain from blood (Acts 15:28, 29).'

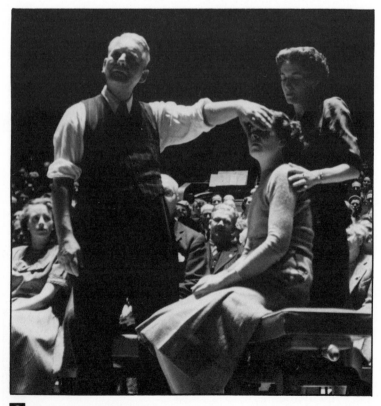

C Faith healer at work.

Justice is our concern

FIGHT WORLD POVERTY

The Brandt Commission Report highlighted the fact that the world's trade and banking systems are unjust to the poor in the Third World.

Our God is a God of Justice, Christians should therefore be committed to the struggle to change these systems.

That is why the major churches, Christian Aid, Tear Fund and Cafod encourage their supporters to join the World Development Movement and campaign to get Britain to change those policies that prevent development in the Third World.

In 1981, the WDM organized the 10,000 strong Mass Lobby of Parliament in May, a nation-wide series of public meetings, and a massive letter-writing campaign to MPs, urging the Government to change its policies towards the Third World.

Must I bother with politics?

The changes needed to fight world poverty require political solutions. Avoiding this area means giving approval to the present unjust system and ignoring God's command that justice is done.

Isn't giving money enough?

It is of course vital to support the work of the aid agencies who do projects in the Third World, but that on its own is not enough. We must actively campaign for just structures in God's world and you can do that by joining WDM.

D From a publicity leaflet by the World Development Movement, an organization supported by some of the most important Christian charity organizations.

A doctor writing in the 'American Journal of Obstetrics and Gynecology' acknowledged: 'There is no doubt that the situation where you [the surgeon] are operating without the possibility of transfusion tends to improve your surgery. You are a little bit more aggressive in clamping every bleeding vessel. All types of surgery can be performed successfully without blood transfusions. This includes open-heart operations, brain surgery and the amputation of limbs.'

Wordbox

status rank or position
resolution decision
Brandt Commission a group set up to discuss world problems to try to persuade important people about an issue
aid agencies organizations for helping the world's needy people.

Questions

1 Look at photograph **B**.
   a What sort of things is the 'traditional' African doctor selling?
   b What advantages might his medicine have over modern scientific medicine?
   c According to document **A**, how is 'traditional' medicine thought of in Africa? Support your answer with a quotation from **A**.
   d Does photograph **B** support what document **A** says about the importance of this kind of medicine in Africa?
2 a Look at photograph **C**. How is the patient being healed?
   b What might some modern doctors think of the method of healing shown in photograph **C**?
3 What do you think is meant in leaflet **D** by the 'present unjust system', and how does the leaflet suggest that Christians should change it?
4 Read the quotes from the Jehovah's Witnesses. Blood transfusions seem to be a good idea. So why does it make sense to the Jehovah's Witnesses not to give blood? Give reasons for your answer.
5 Compare photograph **C** with the medieval picture of the healing of Naaman (page 98). What similarity do you notice?

War and medicine

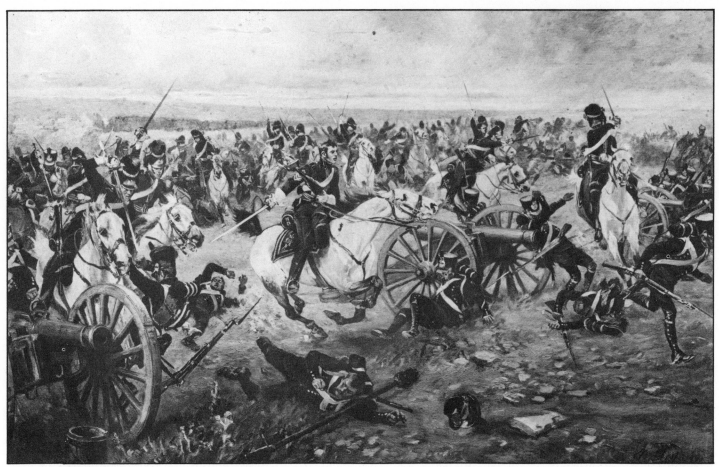

A Waterloo, 1815, by Henri Duprey.

One of the times when medical help is most needed is during wartime. But when we see an artist's impression of war it is like that shown in picture **A**. It was not until the invention of photography that accurate pictures of wars could be mass produced. Even then only certain pictures were allowed to be published.

In all wars the wounded soldiers have suffered a lot. For example, at the battle of Gettysburg, in the American Civil War, 33 000 soldiers were wounded and 7000 died. However, the way they were looked after depended on the army they were in and what people thought about war in those times.

It is not necessarily true that the treatment of soldiers always improved through time. How have wars affected medicine?

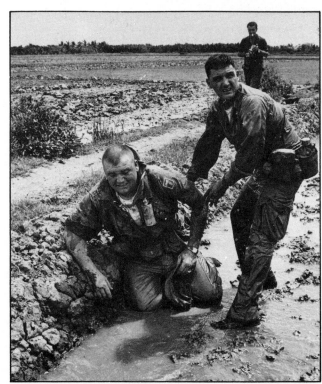

B The stark reality of Vietnam.

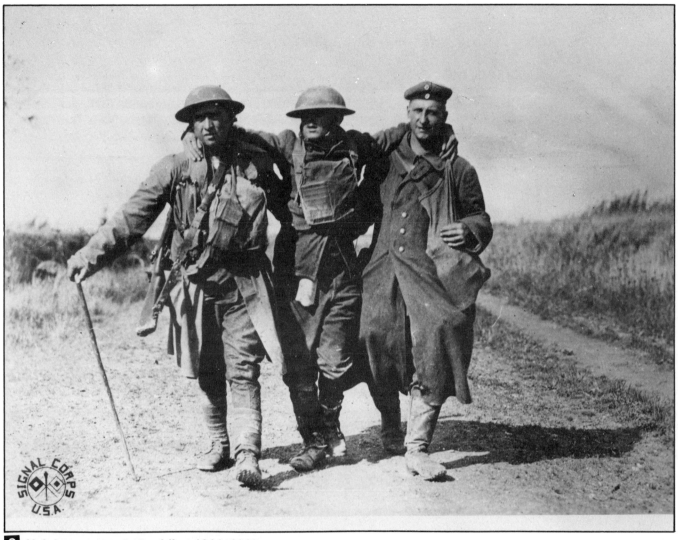

C Helping a wounded soldier, 1914–1918.
The soldier on the left is an American, the soldier on the right is German.

Questions

1 Look at picture **A**. What impression of Waterloo has the artist given?
2 What differences are there between **A** and **B**?
3 How might pictures **A**, **B** and **C** be useful to the historian? Explain your answer.
4 How do you think the following developments might have changed the way people think about war:
   a newspapers
   b photography
   c T.V.?
5 Pictures like **C** were not often allowed to be printed in newspapers. Why not?

6 Copy and complete the chart below as you read through the units on war.

Ways in which wars help medical progress	Ways in which wars hinder (hold back) medical progress
Accurate pictures of casualties gave doctors valuable information about how to treat the wounded.	Lots of people suffer. At Gettysburg in the American Civil War, 33 000 were wounded.

War and transport

Before the wounded can be treated they must be taken quickly from the battlefield. This was not always an easy job. In the Middle Ages men would be left to die where they fell unless their friends carried them away. Earlier the Romans did have special soldiers to help the wounded, and from about the end of the 18th century most armies had medical orderlies whose job it was to help the casualties get to a doctor or surgeon. Unfortunately, this system did not work very well because there were always many more wounded than there were helpers, so army doctors began to look for a solution to this problem.

During the Napoleonic Wars (1789–1815), a French doctor called Baron Dominique Larrey came up with a solution. He designed a light ambulance wagon which brought the wounded to field hospitals where they were treated.

Larrey's ambulance wagon worked quite well and soon the idea was being copied by other armies. During the Crimean War (1853–1856) the armies all had horse-drawn wagons but, because of the conditions on the battlefield, they could not always be used.

B **Surgeon-General Hammond of the Union (Northern) army in the American Civil War (1862–1865), writing after the battle of Bull Run (20 August 1862).**

"

The frightful state of disorder existing in the arrangements for removing the wounded from the field of battle, the lack of ambulances, organization, and the drunkenness and incompetency of the drivers, the total absence of ambulance attendants, are now working their results. . . Wounded remain on the battlefield. Many have died of starvation, many more will die. . . of exhaustion, and all have endured torments which might have been avoided.

"

A Dr Larrey's flying ambulance, 1797.

C American ambulances in France at a dressing station in the First World War (1914–1918).

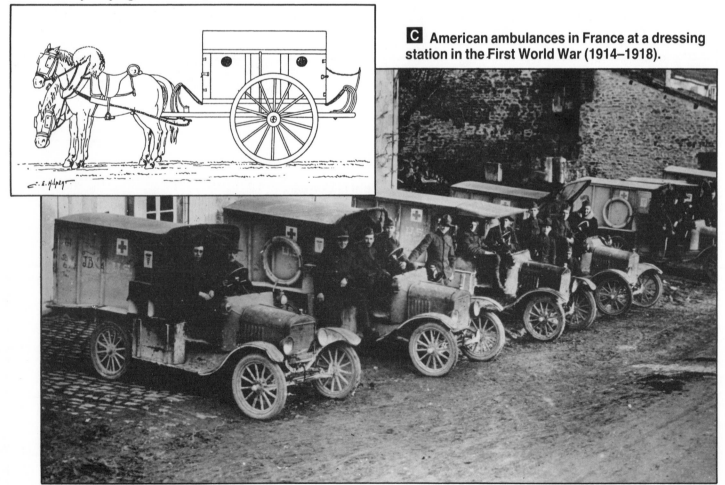

Since the 1800s there have been great changes in methods of transportation. During the First World War (1914–1918) trains were used to transport injured soldiers back to hospitals which were a long way from the battlefield. But advances in technology did not necessarily make it easier for the wounded to be taken from the battlefields, especially when these were as muddy as those of the First World War. The Second World War (1939–1945) saw the development of aircraft as a means of transporting the wounded from the front line to hospitals hundreds of miles away. However, aircraft need runways, and it was only when helicopters came into general use that casualties could be taken directly from almost any battlefield straight to the hospital. In the Falklands War the wounded men could be taken by helicopter to ships waiting nearby which had been converted into hospitals.

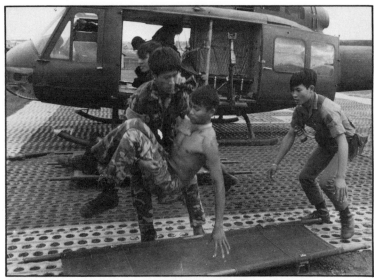

D Vietnam wounded are taken from a helicopter, 1969.

Wordbox

orderlies helped doctors in the army
incompetency uselessness
endured gone through

Questions

1 Copy and complete the chart using pictures **A**, **C** and **D**.
2 Read document **B**. Do you think medical services have improved much since Larrey's time or not? Support your answer with a quotation from document **B**?

War	Middle Ages 1100-1500 (paragraph 1)	Napoleonic Wars 1790-1815 (picture **A**)	First World War 1914-1918 (picture **C**)	Vietnam War 1969 (picture **D**
a How were the wounded soldiers taken off the battlefield?				
b Roughly how many people can be taken in this way?				
c How fast is this method of transport?				
d How well and how comfortably could soldiers be treated?				
e On the way to hospital, under what sort of battlefield conditions can this type of movement be used?				

War and the wounded

Wars wound more soldiers than they kill. The injuries depend on the sorts of weapons used in battle. If the medical services are good, then more soldiers have a chance of survival. Napier, a historian of the Napoleonic Wars (in the early 19th century) commented that the remarkable work of the medical officers might be said to have saved the day at the battle of Vittoria (1813), for their exertions had added between 4000 and 5000 men to Wellington's army without whom Wellington might well have lost.

A Extract from 'The Roman Imperial Army', G Webster (1979).

"

There is a scene on a monument called Trajan's Column showing a wounded legionary sitting on a rock being attended by an orderly who appears to be carrying out an examination. Next to him is an auxiliary having a thigh wound bandaged. The main task of the field orderlies was to patch up the wounds and get the men into a hospital as soon as possible. The main tasks of the medic would have been the cleaning and stitching of gashes and swords cuts and extraction of missiles.

"

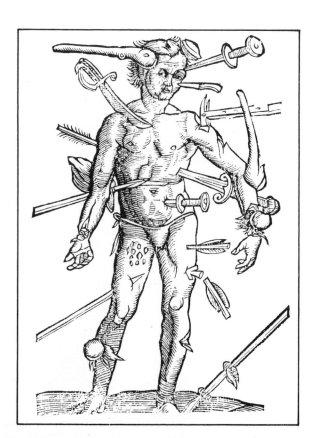

In the unit on medieval surgery we saw that Roman methods of dealing with the wounded were not continued. The injured often had to look after themselves, or suffer the pain of hot tar, burning oil and the cautery iron being put on to their wounds. We saw that Paré used a different method – a soothing ointment and some ligatures – which seemed to be more successful. However even while Paré was alive we find this comment:

C Description of the quality of surgeons, by the surgeon Thomas Gales in the 16th century.

"

I remember the war at Montremil, 1544, when there was a great rabble that called themselves surgeons. Some were tinkers, others were shoe repairers. The general became suspicious about the large number of people that died of small wounds. He sent for me and for other surgeons so as to find out how these people had died. Was it because of their wounds, or because of the lack of knowledge of the surgeons? We searched the camp and demanded to know if these men really were surgeons. They showed us their surgical equipment. Grease for horses' heels, shoemakers' wax, rusty pans. When threatened by the general to be hanged, this rabble confessed their true occupations.

"

However, 300 years later, people were still worried about the treatment of the wounded, and at last something was done.

D From 'Soldiers', a television programme, 1985.

"

Sickened by the sight of casualties at the battle of Solferino in 1859, the Swiss businessman Henri Dunant swore to change the habits of nations. What shocked Dunant was that many of the wounded still lay out for days, as they always had. The others were cared for in ramshackle field hospitals whose doctors were overwhelmed by the scale of their task. His campaign brought about the first Geneva convention, which set up the Red Cross, an organization which treated the wounded of both sides.

"

B (Left) A 'wound man' from a book published in 1593.

Infections from wounds were the most serious problems with which war doctors had to deal. Although progress was being made in the early 20th century towards the production of drugs to fight this kind of infection, it was not until 1943 that penicillin was mass produced by the American chemical industry to meet the huge demands of the Second World War. Although penicillin was a very powerful drug it didn't cure all infections caused by wounds. Another drug had been developed in the 1930s called sulphonamide. Like penicillin, it was mass produced so that by 1943 all American soldiers carried with them a packet containing 12 sulphonamide tablets and a small amount of powder for smearing on any wound.

In England, newly discovered blood transfusions increased enormously the chances of survival. By the time of the Second World War, blood transfusions had improved so much that it was possible to do them on the battlefield.

Because more people recovered from their wounds it meant that, even if you lost a limb in war, you still had a good chance of survival. This meant that there was more demand for all sorts of artificial limbs. At first they were made out of wood. Later, plastics were used.

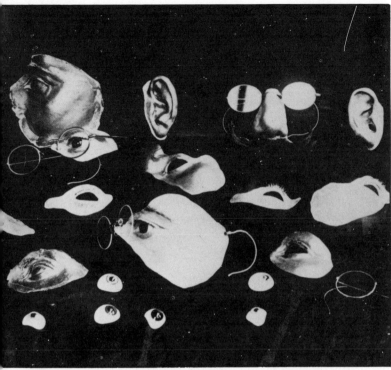

E Plates for First World War soldiers with facial injuries.

Wordbox

auxiliary assistant
medic medical helper on a battlefield
extraction pulling out
missile weapon sent through the air
ligature something used to tie up the veins to stop the bleeding
tinkers travellers selling small goods
ramshackle untidy mess
convention agreement

Questions

1 Read document **A**. What sort of wounds did soldiers get in Roman times and how were they dealt with?
2 Look at picture **B**. List the wounds that soldiers got. What differences do you notice from Roman times?
3 If you were a wounded soldier, when would you prefer to be treated and why:
   a Roman times, or
   b Middle Ages?
   Explain your answer.

4 Read document **D**. Why do you think the Red Cross was an improvement on earlier ways of dealing with war wounded?
5 Look at picture **E**.
   a What materials seem to have been used?
   b How successful might they have been?
6 Add the examples from these two pages to the chart started on page 103.

War and people

Each war brings new medical problems. Of all the new weapons in the First World War (1914–1918) which tested the skills of doctors, gas, the 'devil's breath' was the most feared.

A Extract from BBC TV programme 'Soldiers', 1985. The soldier from the First World War remembers a gas attack.

"

It killed thousands and when you'd seen the others you thought, I hope it doesn't get me like it got them. Those who saw the state the gas victims were in would rather have got shot through the heart straight away than get over it. It was horrible. As we were running into the gas one man suggested tying a wet handkerchief round your nose and mouth. Then our officer said that'd be no use at all. He said it's chlorine gas and the antidote to chlorine is salammoniac. We can't get the salammoniac, the nearest we can get to it is your pee. So what we did was tear our shirts and urinate on them. Nobody would help you because they wanted their own shirt.

"

The First and Second World Wars were different from other wars in history because they affected everybody in the countries at war in some way or other, as we see in these documents.

Another feature of European wars in the 20th century has been rationing. This is a method introduced by governments to make sure that people have a fair amount of food.

C Extract from 'A History of Medicine' by Brian Inglis, 1965.

"

The only time when preventive medicine really flourished was during wars, when the need to prevent people from falling sick, as distinct from curing them when they did, was urgent. It took conscription in the First World War to reveal the depressingly low physical standards of soldiers in many countries; and this was to lead to greater attention later being paid to physical check-ups and better school meals.

"

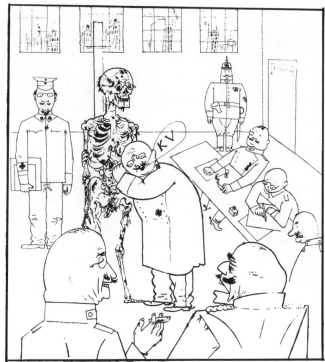

B German cartoon about the health of a new soldier who has been conscripted into the German army in the First World War. (KV in German is short for 'fit for active service'.)

D From 'Life in Wartime Britain' by E R Chamberlain, 1972.

"

It is probable that the very poor ate better during the war than at any period before. Feeding the hungry was no longer a charity but part of the 'war effort'. The numbers of school children receiving free or heavily subsidised meals soared: their parents could get balanced meals at proportionately less than they had paid for the bread, marge, and fish and chips diet of pre-war years. The vast majority of the population kept good health.

"

Wordbox

chlorine a yellowish gas
antidote something that stops a poison
salammoniac ammonium chloride
conscripted made to go in the army
CND Campaign for Nuclear Disarmament

Of all the weapons developed for use in warfare, the atomic bomb presents medicine with the largest number of problems. It has obvious immediate effects, but even 40 years after the dropping of the first atomic bomb, people are still dying from it. These documents give different points of view about the chances of survival.

E **Leon Brittan MP, 'The Times', 22 December 1980.**

"

What I have always said is that nuclear war would lead to appalling results and millions of people being killed. But, however horrible, much could be done to save lives. Outside the immediate target area even the simplest ideas in 'Protect and Survive', the government booklet, would lead to a massive reduction in casualties.

"

'Protect and Survive' is a booklet produced by the British government. It advises people how to survive an atomic explosion.

F **Statement issued by the 30th Pugwash Conference on Science and World Affairs. Quoted in 'Sanity', the magazine of CND, April/May 1981.**

"

Effective civil defence against nuclear attack is impossible . . . in sum, there are no defences against the lethal effects of nuclear weapons, and there is no effective treatment for those who initially survive a nuclear attack.

"

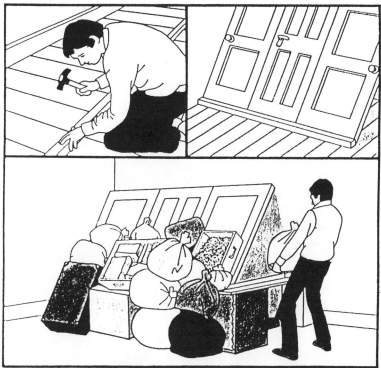

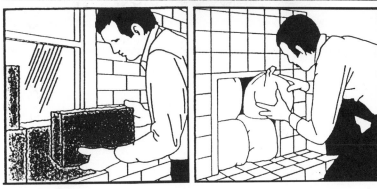

G Pictures from the British government booklet 'Protect and Survive'.

Questions

1 Look at cartoon **B**. What does the cartoonist think about conscription?
2 How did wars encourage the improvement of the health of poor people? Give examples from documents **C** and **D**.
3 What are the advantages and disadvantages of cartoons as a source of evidence (picture **B**)?
4 What advice is being given in the booklet 'Protect and Survive' as seen in picture **G**?
5 What are the differences between documents **E** and **F**? Explain why they disagree.
6 Add examples from this page to the chart (question 1) on page 105.
7 'War leads and medicine follows.' What do you think this means? Support your answer with evidence from any of the war chapters.

Alexander Fleming and Elizabeth Blackwell

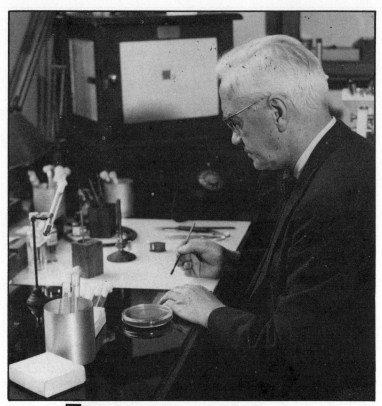

A Alexander Fleming (1881–1955) in his laboratory.

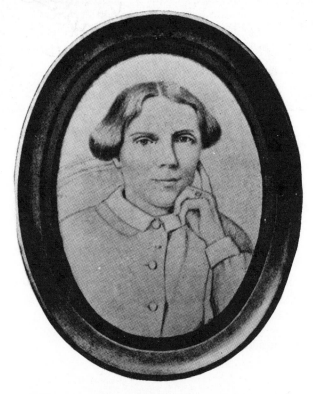

B Dr Elizabeth Blackwell (1821–1910).

Alexander Fleming

Penicillin has been called the wonder drug of the 20th century. It has saved millions of people's lives and relieved a lot of pain. The man who discovered penicillin was Alexander Fleming. He was a Scottish biochemist who had seen in the First World War how thousands of men had died terrible, painful deaths from infection. He decided to do something about this when he left the army. For 10 years after the war he carried out scientific experiments in his laboratory.

In this laboratory Fleming grew bacteria on small plates and tested them to see if they killed germs. Although he tried thousands of plates, none of them seemed to work. Then, one day in 1928, just before his summer holidays, he began some more experiments. Because it was so hot he left the window open. He went away. When he returned to the laboratory he quickly checked the plates to see what had happened to them. He was not very hopeful. Nothing special seemed to have happened to them and he decided to wash them up and start again. Suddenly, to his surprise, he noticed a huge blob on one of the plates. The blob seemed to have killed the germs around it. This was just what he had been looking for!

He grew some more of the mould, called Penicillium Notatum, and realized that it killed many different germs. However, he found it difficult to grow large amounts of the mould, so he couldn't easily do experiments to prove how successful it was. Not much was done to develop it into a drug until the outbreak of the Second World War (1939–1945). Once again, huge numbers of soldiers died of infections, but the few who were treated with 'penicillin' quickly recovered. This encouraged the American and British governments to organize the mass production of the drug.

Elizabeth Blackwell

The first woman to get a degree in medicine from an American university was Elizabeth Blackwell. The way in which she got started in her medical career was unusual.

Women were not allowed to enter American universities to study medicine in the middle of the 19th century. However, Elizabeth Blackwell was a very determined person. Even though her application to study medicine was turned down by many universities; she did not give up. Finally she applied to the Geneva College of Medicine, New York. The dean of the university told his students that if they all voted to admit her he would allow her to study at the university. He was sure that they would vote to reject her, because a woman's place was thought to be in the home in those days.

However, his students thought he was joking, so they decided to go along with the joke and voted unanimously to admit Miss Blackwell to the university. As soon as she heard of their decision, Elizabeth insisted that the dean keep his word and let her start her studies. The joke that went wrong had given a woman the chance to study medicine at last. From then on there were many difficulties, but Elizabeth overcame them and eventually gained her degree. Many people in the town thought the idea of a woman studying medicine was so horrible that they refused to talk to her. Some people tried to get her banned from the lectures on the body, because they thought it unsuitable for a woman to know about such a subject. However, Elizabeth Blackwell was so hard working that she won the respect of her fellow students and, in the end, they insisted that she be allowed to go to the lectures. She got top marks in the exams and was presented with her degree in 1849.

There were still many battles to be fought in the struggle for equal rights in the medical profession, but Elizabeth Blackwell had brought nearer the time when universities all over the world would accept women as medical students.

The Tamil workers
The Tamils are a group of people who come from India and Sri Lanka. About 100 years ago, some of these Tamil workers were taken thousands of miles away to work in the fields in Malaya. The Tamils had a custom that water should be brought into their house and used only once a day. The Malayan people who worked in the same fields brought barrels of water into their houses and kept the water there for days. Mosquitoes could breed easily in these barrels and spread terrible diseases like dengue and malaria. Nobody at this time knew what caused these diseases, but far fewer Tamils died from them because of their custom.

The marmot
Picture **C** shows marmots feeding. The marmots are members of the rodent family. Some of the nomadic tribes of China believed that their relatives and friends were reincarnated as marmots. So marmots were treated with special care and respect. The tribes kept their distances from marmots. Scientists today know that the marmot can carry plague germs. So, even though they didn't know about germs, the tribes avoided catching the plague!

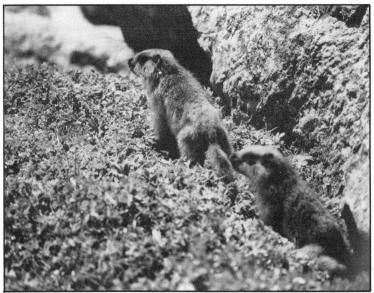

C The long-tailed marmot.

Wordbox

unanimously   agreed by everyone
dengue   a fever with very painful swellings
reincarnated   came back to life

Questions

1 What do we mean by the word 'chance'?
2 Choose one of these stories:
  a Dr Elizabeth Blackwell,
  b the marmot, or
  c the Tamil workers.
    (i) Explain why chance was important in this story.
    (ii) Describe what other factors were important in these stories (e.g. religion).
3 Write a few sentences to explain how the following factors helped in the development of penicillin:
  a the First and Second World Wars,
  b scientific methods,
  c chance, and
  d governments.
4 Which of the four factors in question 3 do you think was the most important, and why?

Check your chronology

When we use the word 'chronology' we are talking about the idea of time – and of getting things in the right order. It is important to know what happened in the past and also when it happened. Put these important people and events in the right order. Use the contents page and the timeline (page 124) to help you. Where there are question marks you have to fill in the missing information.

Name	Historical period or people (e.g. Romans, Renaissance etc.)	Why person was important
1 **?**	**?**	He was a Scottish bacteriologist who accidentally discovered penicillin when he noticed an unusual green mould on a dish in his laboratory. It turned out to be the substance from which was made the pain-killing drug which helped millions of people.
2 **Hippocrates**	Ancient Greece	**?**
3 **?**	Egyptians	A god that scared away the evil spirits that were thought to cause disease.
4 **Joseph Lister**	**?**	**?**
5 **?**	– **?**	He became professor of Anatomy at Padua University. He took bodies of executed criminals from the scaffold, so that he could learn about the body. The Pope had forbidden human dissection in 1300, so progress could be made only by going against the church's law. He proved by experiment and observation that Galen's ideas about the shape of the **?** and the ribs were wrong. His book on anatomy called **?** was part of a revolution in art and science. Many people read it because of the discovery of **?**
6 **Robert Koch**	Industrial Revolution	**?**
7 **Ambroise Paré**	Renaissance	**?**
8 **Wilhelm Roentgen**		He was a Dutch professor who carried out experiments using a long glass tube, called a cathode ray tube. When he passed electricity through the tube he found that he could make a picture on a specially treated piece of paper. This was useful for medicine because **?**

REVISION SECTION

Name	Historical period or people (e.g. Romans, Renaissance etc.)	Why person was important
9 **?**	**?**	He was a French scientist whose discovery led to the development of the **?** theory of disease – perhaps the most important medical discovery ever. Using microscope technology and scientific experiments he discovered microbes in wine and eventually found the germs that caused diseases which previously had killed large numbers of people. Once the cause had been identified it became possible to develop **?** against these infectious diseases.
10 **?**	Renaissance/Industrial Revolution	He was an English country doctor who observed that milkmaids didn't get smallpox. He put forward the idea that perhaps these milkmaids didn't get smallpox because they had got a protecting disease from the cows they worked with. He tested out this idea by **?** This was found to be a successful way of stopping smallpox.
11 **?**	**?**	He was a surgeon to the gladiators and to the emperors. He made detailed drawings of the body and his ideas on anatomy were accepted as the truth for **?** years after his death. However, because human dissection was forbidden, he could dissect only animals, so there were limits to what he could find out about.
12 **Imhotep**	**?**	He was probably a pharaoh's physician who was good at his job. Later he came to be worshipped as the god of **?**
13 **?**	Industrial Revolution	He was Professor of Midwifery at Edinburgh. He saw the pain women went through in childbirth and looked for a way of relieving it. One evening he and his colleagues experimented with **?**. They sniffed it and fell unconscious. By demonstrating the use of anaesthetics he had helped bring surgery into the modern age. Longer, more complicated and less painful operations were possible.
14 **?**	Industrial Revolution	He was an English civil servant who produced a report about **?** in Britain. He criticized governments for not doing enough to clean up towns. He suggested important changes. Some of these ideas were ignored. Only when **?** epidemics hit the country was he taken seriously.
15 **Sir William Harvey**	Renaissance	**?**
16 **?**	**?**	He was worshipped as the god of healing. Patients came to his temple at **?** in the hope that they would be cured by faith healing. They took exercise and rested at a sort of building at the temple, called the **?** At night the patient was healed by the holy snake, accompanied by the god's daughters, Hygeia and Panacea.

Understanding change

Things change in history at different times for different reasons. To try to understand how and why things changed in the history of medicine, look at these ideas and find examples from what you've studied.

1 Sometimes there are dramatic turning points in history, for example, the beginnings of space flight.
Find examples to show dramatic turning points in the history of medicine

a *CAUSE AND CURE*	Hippocrates brought about a more scientific approach to medicine. Instead of blaming gods and spirits for disease, Hippocrates showed that disease has 'natural' causes and cures.
b *SURGERY*	**?**
c *PUBLIC HEALTH*	**?**
d *ANATOMY AND PHYSIOLOGY*	Vesalius showed, by scientific experiment and by the dissection of human corpses, that some of Galen's ideas about the structure of the human body were completely wrong. These ideas had been accepted and unchallenged for over a thousand years. Vesalius' discoveries led to a greater understanding of the body.

2 Sometimes things don't change for a long period of time. For example, for thousands of years man travelled by horse (or other animals) and only much later did he develop mechanically-powered transport.
Find examples from the history of medicine to show things not changing for a long period of time.

a *CAUSE AND CURE*	Spiritual ideas about the cause and cure of disease have lasted from prehistoric times up until today.
b *SURGERY*	The red-hot cautery iron was used for hundred of years as a way of stopping the flow of blood before less cruel methods were eventually found.
c *PUBLIC HEALTH*	**?**
d *ANATOMY AND PHYSIOLOGY*	**?**

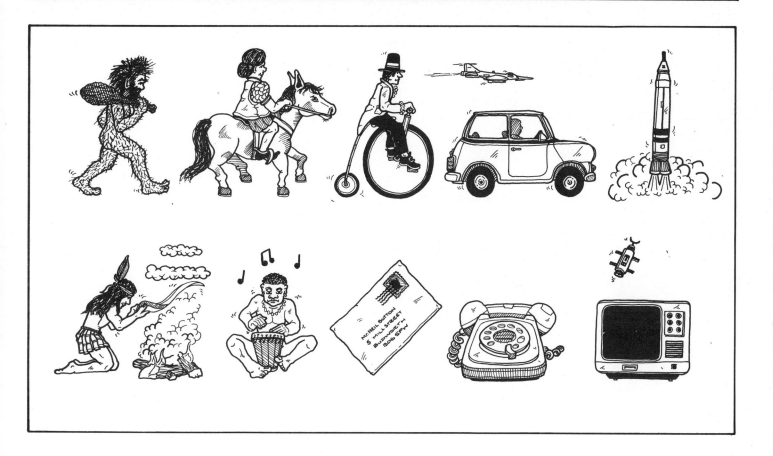

3 Sometimes things get worse, not better, over the years. For example, the Romans built superb roads but in later years the roads fell into decay, and in the Middle Ages the roads were very much worse than they had been in Roman times.
Find examples from the history of medicine to show things getting worse, not better.

---

a *CAUSE AND CURE*   **?**

---

b *SURGERY*   The Romans had military hospitals and looked after their wounded soldiers very well. Medieval surgeons had no such facilities – indeed, they had to operate on soldiers in terrible conditions, out in the open air of the battlefield.

---

c *PUBLIC HEALTH*   **?**

---

d *ANATOMY AND PHYSIOLOGY*   The Egyptians had an idea of the workings of the heart, but after the collapse of the Egyptian empire things got generally worse, until the discoveries made by Harvey about blood circulation in the 17th century.

Factors of change

Change often comes about because different 'factors' work together to bring it about. For example, we all depend on the society in which we live. Take the story of a plane which crashed on a desert island. One of the survivors is a doctor. Despite his personal qualities and his knowledge, he might not be able to treat all the survivors because he lacks a number of things such as technical equipment, communications, and people with other skills, such as nurses.

A diagram may help to explain how many factors contribute to medical advancement. Take the examples of Louis Pasteur's and Robert Koch's fight against infectious disease. We could help explain why their fight against infectious diseases was won by showing some of the many factors which played their part.

The battle against infectious diseases

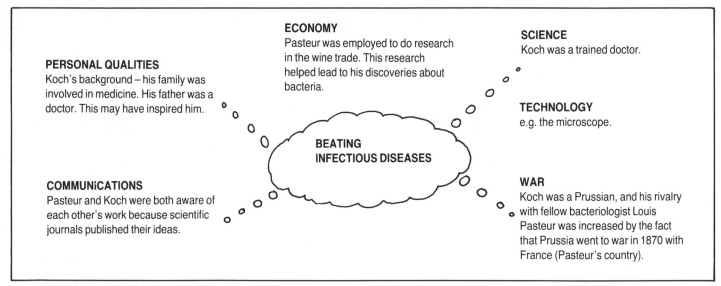

ECONOMY
Pasteur was employed to do research in the wine trade. This research helped lead to his discoveries about bacteria.

SCIENCE
Koch was a trained doctor.

PERSONAL QUALITIES
Koch's background – his family was involved in medicine. His father was a doctor. This may have inspired him.

TECHNOLOGY
e.g. the microscope.

BEATING INFECTIOUS DISEASES

COMMUNICATIONS
Pasteur and Koch were both aware of each other's work because scientific journals published their ideas.

WAR
Koch was a Prussian, and his rivalry with fellow bacteriologist Louis Pasteur was increased by the fact that Prussia went to war in 1870 with France (Pasteur's country).

Other factors – like chance and religion – did not play a very important part in the fight against infectious diseases, but they were important in other parts of medical history.

1 Draw a similar diagram (the outline is provided) to show the factors which help explain Vesalius' contribution to the growth of new ideas about anatomy. Copy the titles and write a sentence to explain *each* factor.

Vesalius and new ideas about anatomy

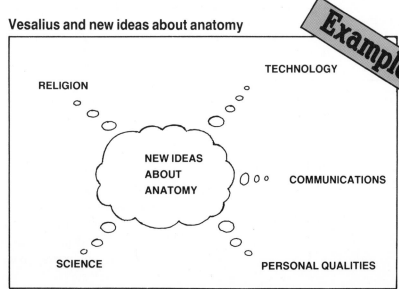

RELIGION

TECHNOLOGY

NEW IDEAS ABOUT ANATOMY

COMMUNICATIONS

SCIENCE

PERSONAL QUALITIES

Example

Change comes about for many reasons, or 'factors', such as the discoveries made by 'great' people. For example, the Wright brothers' successfully flying the aeroplane. However, in what ways were these people 'great'? Why was it Paré that made great surgical discoveries rather than anybody else? What personal qualities did people like Paré have?

2 Find examples from the history of medicine to show the personal qualities of great people.

a *CAUSE AND CURE*	
b *SURGERY*	James Simpson was strong enough to stand up to the opposition of the Church to his use of chloroform as an anaesthetic. He also showed that he was prepared to take risks in experimenting with chloroform on himself!
c *PUBLIC HEALTH*	Edwin Chadwick was dedicated, patient, hard working and determined. He had to put up with his ideas being ignored for years, as well as the opposition of wealthy people who didn't want to pay for the public health reforms he suggested.
d *ANATOMY AND PHYSIOLOGY*	

Change doesn't just come about because of personal qualities; it has to do with other factors in the times in which people live. For example, Stephenson couldn't have made the steam locomotive if someone else hadn't invented the steam engine. Even 'great' people depend on other things to make their discoveries. Hippocrates seems to have been an intelligent person (he has been called the 'Father of Medicine'), but he never discovered germs, which are the most important things to know about in finding cures. He couldn't do this because of the times in which he lived. For example, the Greeks had no microscopes.

Paré was a great man who made important contributions to surgery, but he couldn't completely solve the three important problems facing the surgeon – pain, bleeding and infection. Why not?

3 Find reasons or 'factors' to explain why Paré couldn't solve these problems.
  a Pain: even in Paré's time, scientists did not have the technical knowledge to make anaesthetics like laughing gas or chloroform.
  b Infection: He couldn't solve this problem because . . .

Going to the doctor through the ages

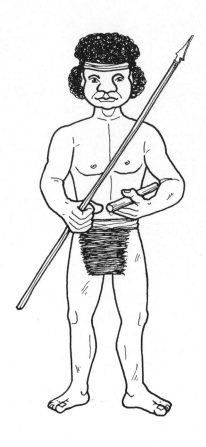

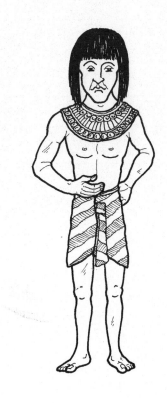

1 Here is an aborigine. He has a wide variety of medical problems. What you must do is suggest how he ought to be treated. The suggestions you make *must* be the ones an aborigine doctor would have made.

Copy the picture, the problems and your answers into your books or folders. Use pages 8–9 to help you.

a He has burnt his leg in a fire.
b He has broken his arm.
c The man complains of bad headaches. What might have caused them?
d Would you dance and chant to cure the man? If so, why?
e He has cut his hand.
f Of all your cures, which ones are you confident will work? Why?

2 The Pharaoh of Egypt is ill. You have been called in to cure him. How would you treat him if you were an Egyptian doctor?

Use pages 12–13 to help you. Copy the picture, the problems and your answers into your books or folders.

a If he dies, what are you going to do with the body?
b He's got a boil on his bottom. How will you treat it?
c He has broken his arm. What will you do?
d He complains of a pain in the stomach. Explain how it may have come about.
e He thinks Bes has put a spell on him. Can you get rid of it?
f He is going blind. Are you able to help him?
g Of all your cures, which ones are you confident will work? Explain why.

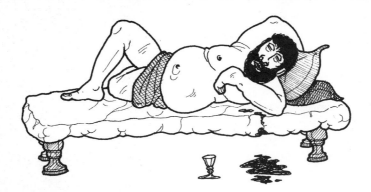

3 Here is a sick Roman. What you must do is suggest how he might be treated.

Answer the questions as if you were a Roman doctor. Use pages 20–21 to help you. Remember the Romans followed some Greek ideas.

a It is the height of summer and you are called to the home of a very sick man (a merchant). What things would you do first?

b He is hot, sweating, vomiting, and complains about having pains in his stomach. What is wrong with him?

c He is rather fat and a bit smelly, with bad teeth. He says that his servants carry him wherever he wants to go. Recommend a healthier way of life for him.

d If he asks for some kind of treatment, which place would you suggest he goes to?

e If he gets well he will make an offering to a god. Which would you suggest?

f If he breaks his arm, how would you treat him?

g If you failed to get rid of the man's fever but mended his arm, how would you explain your success at one medical problem and failure with another?

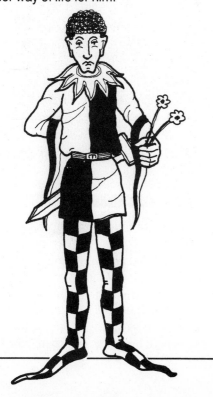

4 Sir Percival has got a few problems. If you were a doctor in the Middle Ages, how would you treat him?

Look at pages 24–25 to help you.

a He says that he has got a fever. How will you check this?

b Will you suggest flebotomy? If so, what will you do?

c He looks a rich man. How might this affect any herbal remedy you might give him?

d Suggest what he needs to do to stay healthy.

e How can you check your diagnosis and treatments?

f He is very religious. How will this affect what you say about his illness and how you will treat it?

Making judgements and comparisons

Some factors are more important than others. Which of the following was most important? For each of questions 1–4, copy out the list of reasons, or factors, in order of importance, and explain your choice.

1 Why didn't the aborigines make progress in medicine?

a	*Economy*	Nomadic lifestyle.
b	*Communications*	No contact with outside world.
c	*Religion*	Superstitious explanations of the world.
d	*Technology*	Stone-age tools.

2 Why were the Egyptians able to improve knowledge about the heart?

a *Economy* — The Egyptians were farmers. This gave them a more settled way of life and allowed them to live in one place. Because they didn't have to spend all their time hunting, they had time to educate themselves in new skills.

b *Communications* — The Egyptians traded with other countries so they picked up useful ideas and new information.

c *Religion* — They believed in life after death, and mummified important people. So as to preserve the bodies of the dead they had to find out more about the heart and the other organs of the body.

d *Technology* — To build pyramids they needed better technology. They made bronze tools, which were an improvement on what had been produced before.

3 Why was Roman public health so good?

a *Economy* — The Romans had a huge system of slave labour. This helped them carry out large building projects, such as the construction of roads, aqueducts etc. Slavery left Romans free to learn new skills.

b *Chance* — The Romans didn't know that germs caused disease but they built their towns in hygienic places, away from swamps and other dangerous positions.

c *War* — The Romans conquered and controlled a huge empire with a strong army. To win battles the army needed to be fit and healthy. So the Romans provided clean, well designed houses, good sewers, baths and toilets, and also battlefield hospitals.

d *Technology* — They had iron tools and well designed equipment which helped them improve their building skills.

4 Why was Jenner able to improve the understanding of infectious diseases?

a *Science* — Jenner was a trained doctor who had been treating smallpox sufferers for a long time.

b *Communications* — Better communications allowed news of a Turkish treatment of smallpox to reach Jenner in England.

c *Chance* — It was a lucky break for Jenner that a dairy maid told him that people who had already had cowpox did not get smallpox.

d *Personal qualities* — Jenner was prepared to take the risk of the vaccination experiment. He was also determined enough to carry on with his work, even when the Royal Society refused to believe his ideas.

Ancient Indian medicine had many things in common with the European medicine we have looked at in this book. In some ways the Indians were more advanced, in others slightly more ignorant. Here are four of the important features of ancient Indian medicine from 2000 BC to 800 BC. This is known as the Vedic period. Compare this with ancient Egypt.

The Vedic period　　　　　　　　　　　　　　　　　　*Ancient Egypt*

The Vedic period	Ancient Egypt
1 Dhanvantari, god of medicine.	?
2 Religious writing containing magical ways to treat diseases.	?
3 Demons were thought to cause disease.	?
4 Herbs recommended in treatments.	?

The Brahmanistic period in Indian history was from 800 BC to 1000 AD.

Below are listed eleven features of life during that period. Compare these with ancient Greece, ancient Rome and the Middle Ages.^

The Brahmanistic period

The Brahmanistic period	Ancient Greece	Ancient Rome	The Middle Ages
1 Caraka and Sustrata (a doctor and a surgeon) were famous for their medical books.			
2 The Hindu religion, India's main religion at the time, did not allow people to cut up bodies.			
3 Hindu religion was very strict about people keeping clean. Bathing, cleaning teeth and washing eyes was very important.			
4 Didn't know very much about how the body worked.			
5 They believed the body was made up of three elements: spirit (or air), phlegm and bile.			
6 They identified 1120 different diseases.			
7 They could inoculate children against smallpox.			
8 They used bleeding to treat patients.			
9 They used herbs, bits of animals and minerals such as lead, copper and gold in their remedies.			
10 Alcohol was used as an anaesthetic.			
11 They were very good at one or two simple surgical operations and could also do basic 'plastic' surgery such as replacing noses!			

Questions

1 Compare each sentence on India with medical ideas from Europe at the same time, and say if they were the same or different. Copy each one down and write your comments about European medicine next to it.

2 From what you have written, do you think Indian medicine was better or worse than European medicine at the same time? Give reasons for your answer.

3 Suggest reasons why Indian medicine and European medicine had so much in common.

Working things out

Seeing people's points of view

In this section there is a number of statements made about people in the past. You have to copy each of the statements and explain whether you think it is true or false. You will get marks for showing that you understand how people in the past may have thought and behaved. Remember that the whole idea is to see that people in the past thought differently from us. Different people living at the same time might not necessarily have agreed with each other. It will be important to look back at the 'Medicine Through Time' section to help you understand the way of life of the people mentioned in the statements. Once again you will get better marks if you find evidence to back up your answers. Remember to look at the Contents page and Index to help you find extra evidence.

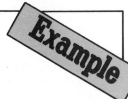

Here is an example. Read this sentence:
'The aborigines of the past had no idea about how to treat disease.'
  In the section about the aborigines (pages 8–9) we looked at evidence like the photograph below.

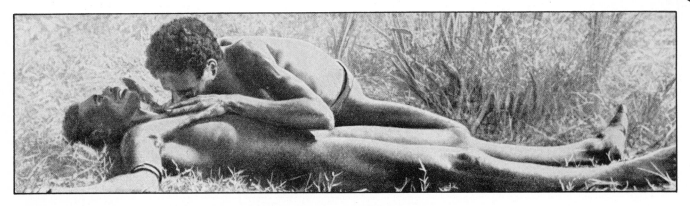

  This evidence suggested that although the aborigines didn't have scientific knowledge, they had treatments which were successful. People believed in the medicine man's power to fight the evil spirits, and many patients were successfully treated by him.

1 Prehistoric people probably thought that trepanning was a sensible idea. (See pages 6–7.)
2 Prehistoric people knew nothing about anatomy. (See pages 6 and 56.)
3 The Egyptians were so interested in religion that it held them back from making advances in science and technology. (See pages 10–13 and page 56.)
4 All Greeks believed in the theory of the four humours and other scientific ideas. (See pages 16–17 and 44–45.)
5 All Greeks were able to follow Hippocrates' programme for health. (See page 17.)
6 Poor people in Rome usually suffered more ill health than the rich. (See pages 66–69.)

7 The medieval peasant had no hope of curing any illness. (See page 76.)
8 Paré's new ideas about surgery made sense to all the people in Renaissance times. (See page 37.)
9 People were quick to accept Jenner's ideas about smallpox. (See pages 47 and 49.)
10 Scientific proof made it easy to get medical ideas accepted in the 19th century. (See pages 39 and 41.)
11 Now germs have been discovered, people agree about what causes disease. (See pages 100–101.)

REVISION SECTION

Solving the problems

Historians make decisions about the past by thinking of ideas and then testing those ideas with historical evidence. We use the word hypothesis to describe these ideas or problems. For example, we can test the idea that:

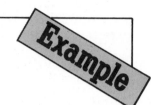

'There is no disease which modern medicine cannot cure.'
In the section about the Welfare State (page 90–91) we looked at evidence like the government leaflet shown below.

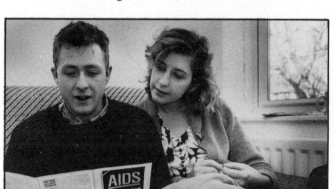

This leaflet suggests that there are in fact some diseases which modern medicine cannot cure. The government found it necessary to send to every house information which warned about the dangers of this deadly disease.

Now have a look at the list of ideas and problems (given below), which you can solve by using your knowledge and this book. Copy the sentences and explain whether you agree or disagree with them. Give reasons for your answers. Marks are given for fitting the best evidence from the book to your answer. The Contents page and the Index will also help you.

1 Scientific ideas about medicine started with the Romans. (See pages 16–17 and 20–21.)
2 Medieval medicine was held back by religion. (See pages 36–37 and 60–61.)
3 Without knowledge of anatomy and physiology there could be no advance in surgery. (See pages 36–37 and 60–61.)
4 The story of X-rays shows that new technology can bring both benefits and problems. (See pages 64–65.)
5 The part played by women in the history of medicine has often been ignored. (See pages 74–81.)
6 Advances made in technology and medicine haven't always been shared out equally throughout the world. (See pages 52–53 and 72–73.)

7 Medieval medicine was more scientific than ancient medicine. (See pages 6–7, 22–23, 34–37 and 56–57.)
8 Surgery was held back by a lack of proper tools until the 20th century. (See pages 34–41.)
9 War was a very important factor in medical change. (See pages 102–109.)
10 The Egyptians were more interested in religion than medicine. (See pages 10–13 and page 56.)
11 The Greeks treated the symptoms of illness and not the causes. (See pages 16–17 and 44–45.)
12 Very important changes in medicine came about during the Renaissance. (See pages 28–29 and 58–63.)
13 The health of the people gets better only when governments get involved in it. (See pages 84–93.)

Timeline

Historical period (Remember, all these dates are approximate)	People	What happened?
Prehistoric peoples **Earlier than about 3000 BC**	No evidence for these individuals	There is little evidence from this period to help us find out about medicine. From what there is we can say they did simple surgical operations like trepanning. We can try to make guesses about prehistoric medicine, but this doesn't really tell us what it was like. Cave paintings tell us about the importance of hunting animals. We don't think that their way of life changed very much over thousands of years.
Ancient Egyptians **3000 BC – 1000 BC**	Imhotep (about 2600 BC)	We have lots more evidence about the Egyptians. They used the River Nile to develop an advanced way of life. Living in cities helped them to develop a wide range of skills, of which medicine was just one. Religion both helped and hindered their medicine. Advances were made in most aspects of medicine.
India and China **3000 BC onwards**		At the same time as the Egyptian civilization, progress was being made in medicine further east, in India and China. The Indians developed a complex civilization which had considerable knowledge of public health, surgery and various other aspects of medicine. Both China and India developed medical ideas that were unknown in Europe until much later.
Greece **800–400 BC**	Asklepios (worshipped about 5000 BC) Hippocrates (about 460 BC)	The Greeks were a prosperous nation of traders who settled in city states and encouraged learning. They developed some important ideas to do with medicine. Some Greeks believed in natural causes for diseases, such as the four humours, while others still believed in gods as the cause and cure of disease.
Romans **400 BC– 400 AD**	Galen (131–201 AD)	The Romans conquered a huge empire with their powerful army and grew rich through farming, slavery and trade. They took many of their ideas from the Greeks. Even their most famous doctor, Galen, was a Greek. They believed in health for all the people and so developed a good public health system. Some of their aqueducts and sewers still survive today. They were good organizers and practical people.

REVISION SECTION

Historical period (Remember, all these dates are approximate)	People	What happened?
Islam **600 AD onwards**	Avicenna (980–1037 AD) Rhazes (about 860–932 AD)	The Arabs fought many wars with Christian Europe and, as a result, their ideas have not always been well understood in Europe. However, they developed the ideas of the Greeks and Romans in their own way. Their scientific and medical ideas were often more advanced than Christian ones. They had medical schools and knew a lot about health and hygiene.
Middle Ages in Europe **400 AD– 1500 AD**		The Christian church dominated people's ideas during this period. Kings needed the help of the church to rule effectively. Most of the skills, knowledge and technology available were used for religious purposes.
Renaissance in Europe **1500– 1700 AD**	Vesalius (1514–1564) Paré (1510–1590) Harvey (1578–1657)	The word 'Renaissance' means re-birth. Many of the better ideas of ancient civilizations were added to. Printing was invented, which helped spread new ideas much more quickly. Better transport and communications developed. There was greater knowledge about anatomy, physiology and surgery. Technological advances affecting medicine were being made, such as the invention of the microscope. But many epidemic diseases could not be stopped.
Industrial Revolution and modern times **1800 AD to the present day**	Jenner (1749–1823) Pasteur (1822–1895) Simpson (1811–1870) Lister (1827–1912) Nightingale (1820–1910) Koch (1843–1910) Chadwick (1801–1890) Roentgen (1845–1923) Ehrlich (1854–1915) Fleming (1881–1955)	About 200 years ago there was a change in the way things were made. Machines and factories transformed the lives of people in many European countries. This change led to all kinds of developments in communications, transport, government and education. Medicine was just one of the things that was totally changed. The germ theory revolutionized ideas about the cause and cure of disease and brought about major improvements in many other areas of medicine, such as surgery. People benefited as governments became more involved in ensuring the good health of the people. However, not all parts of the world benefited from these changes, and the health of many people in the world is still at risk.

Acknowledgements

The authors and Publishers are grateful to the following for permission to reproduce text extracts, photographs and illustrative material used in this book:

6B The London Museum; 7E Jonathan Cape Ltd.; 8A Axel Poignant Archive; 9B/9C Macmillan & Co; 10B The Mansell Collection; 11C William MacQuitty, Camera Press; 11D The Mansell Collection; 12A William MacQuitty, Camera Press; 12B Photoresources; 14B/15C The Mansell Collection; 19B The Mansell Collection; 20A Batsford Publishers; 21B/21C Hulton Picture Library; 22B The Mansell Collection; 23C/23D Ann Ronan Picture Library; 24A BBC Television; 24B Library of the Wellcome Institute for the History of Medicine; 24E Batsford Publishers; 25F Bodleian Library, Oxford; 26A National Gallery; 27B Windsor Castle, Royal Library, © Her Majesty the Queen.; 28A Hulton Picture Library; 28B Macmillan Publishers Ltd.; 29C Hulton Picture Library; 30A The Tate Gallery, London; 32A Vision International; 32B Daily Telegraph Colour Library; 33C Daily Telegraph Colour Library; 34B Axel Poignant Archive; 35C The Mansell Collection; 36A Bibliotheque Royale, Brussels; 36B Hulton Picture Library; 38B/39C/40A/40B Ann Ronan Picture Library; 41C Vision International; 46A/46C/47F/48C Ann Ronan Picture Library; 49E The Mansell Collection; 50B Longman Group Ltd.; 50C William Heinemann Ltd.; 51E Health Education Council; 52A Vision International; 53B Science Photo Library; 53C The Observer Review; 53D Oxford University Press; 54A Martin Mayer, Network Photographers; 55B-E New Internationalist; 55F New Internationalist/Panos Institute; 55G New Internationalist; 57B The Mansell Collection; 57C Ann Ronan Picture Library; 58A Library for the Wellcome Institute for the History of Medicine; 58B Windsor Castle, Royal Library, © Her Majesty the Queen.; 59C Ann Ronan Picture Library; 60A Ann Ronan Picture Library; 60B Library for the Wellcome Institute for the History of Medicine; 62A Ann Ronan Picture Library; 63B Library for the Wellcome Institute for the History of Medicine; 63C Ann Ronan Picture Library; 64A The Mansell Collection; 65B Library for the Wellcome Institute for the History of Medicine; 65C Vision International; 67C A & C Black (Publishers) Ltd.; 67D Barnaby's Picture Library; 67G The Mansell Collection; 68A Penguin Books Ltd.; 68C Dr Jeremy Burgess/Science Photo Library; 69G The Museum of London; 69H The Weald and Down Open Air Housing Museum; 70A/71F The Mansell Collection; 72B New Internationalist Calendar; 72D World Health Organisation; 73C Sarah Errington, Camera Press; 74A Harry Abrams (Publishing); 74B Hulton Picture Library; 74C Constable Young Books; 74E Oxford University Press; 75F/76A The Mansell Collection; 76B Library of the Wellcome Institute for the History of Medicine; 77C/78A The Mansell Collection; 78B Library for the Wellcome Institute for the History of Medicine; 79C The Mansell Collection; 80A Harry Abrams (Publishing); 80B Imperial War Museum; 80C BPCC Publishing Corporation; 81E Camera Press; 83E Ann Ronan Picture Library; 83F Design Team Partnership; 84A The Mansell Collection; 84D Roger Wood; 85E Imperial War Museum; 86A/87B The Mansell Collection; 88A Library for the Wellcome Institute for the History of Medicine; 89D Basil Blackwell Ltd.; 90A Hulton Picture Library; 91D Geoff Franklin, Network Photographers; 92A The Daily Mail; 92E The Sunday Times; 93B Jake Tebbitt; 94A Hamlyn Group Picture Library; 94B The Reverend L.A.N. Jolly and The Royal Commission on Historical Monuments; 96B Dr Jeremy Burgess/Science Photo Library; 98A British Musuem; 99D The Mansell Collection; 100A The Daily Telegraph; 100B WHO/Paul Almacy; 100C/102A Hulton Picture Library; 102B James Pickerell, Camera Press; 103C Hulton Picture Library; 104C Hulton Picture Library; 105E Normand H. Choiniere, Camera Press; 106A A & C Black (Publishers) Ltd.; 106B Ann Ronan Picture Library; 106D BBC Television; 107E Horace W Nicholls; 108A BBC Television; 108B George Grosz, Museum of Modern Art, N.Y.; 108C Weidenfeld and Nicolson; 109G Controller of Her Majesty's Stationery Office; 109E The Times; 109F Sanity/CND; 110A St. Mary's Hospital; 110B Hulton Picture Library; 111C Heather Angel.

Picture research by David Pratt.

Illustrations by Neil Sutton.

While every effort has been made to trace all copyright holders this has not been possible in every case. The Publishers apologise for any omissions and, if notified, will correct the matter at the next printing.

Index